MESSAGE FROM THE CHAIRPERSON

I am very pleased to publish *Obesity the Policy Challenges- the Report of the National Taskforce on Obesity.*

Obesity is a major public health problem for both Ireland and our European neighbours, and is described by the World Health Organisation as a 'global epidemic'. Approximately 39% of Irish adults are overweight and 18% are obese. Annually, approximately 2,000 premature deaths are attributed to obesity, at an estimated cost, in economic terms, of €4bn to the State.

The taskforce are very concerned that childhood obesity has become the most prevalent childhood disease in Europe. It is estimated that over 300,000 children on the island of Ireland are overweight and obese and this is projected to increase annually by 10,000. It is clear that halting the rise in levels of overweight and obesity presents a major challenge. This can only be done by a concerted effort by everyone to protect future generations from the inevitable premature deaths, ill health, psychosocial problems and the projected adverse economic costs on society that will arise if we do nothing.

This report sets out recommendations on how we can rise to this challenge. In particular I welcome the recommendation that the implementation of the report be characterised by joined-up policy, real practical engagement by the public and private sectors, the avoidance of duplication of effort or cross-purpose approaches, and the harnessing of existing strategies and agencies. I hope that this report will assist those who are involved in developing policy as well as those who plan, manage and deliver services.

As chairman I want to thank the members of the taskforce for their invaluable contributions and for giving freely of their time in finalising this report. Thanks also to all those who made submissions to the taskforce and contributed to the wide consultation process undertaken. I wish to acknowledge the work of the sub-committees and experts who assisted the taskforce. Finally I would like to thank the editorial sub-group who pulled the various strands of the report together and to the Health Promotion Unit of the Department of Health and Children for their vital contribution to our work. I am particularly grateful to Oilbhe O'Donoghue for her support as secretary to the taskforce.

Mr. John Treacy
Chairman

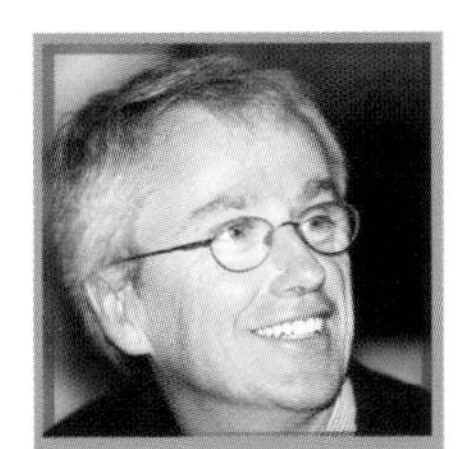

CONTENTS

EXECUTIVE SUMMARY

The prevalence of overweight and obesity has increased with alarming speed over the past twenty years. It has recently been described by the World Health Organisation as a 'global epidemic'. In the year 2000 more than 300 million people worldwide were obese and it is now projected that by 2025 up to half the population of the United States will be obese if current trends are maintained. The disease is now a major public health problem throughout Europe. In Ireland at the present time 39% of adults are overweight and 18% are obese. Of these, slightly more men than women are obese and there is a higher incidence of the disease in lower socio-economic groups.

Most worrying of all is the fact that childhood obesity has reached epidemic proportions in Europe, with body weight now the most prevalent childhood disease. While currently there are no agreed criteria or standards for assessing Irish children for obesity some studies are indicating that the numbers of children who are significantly overweight have trebled over the past decade. Extrapolation from authoritative UK data suggests that these numbers could now amount to more than 300,000 overweight and obese children on the island of Ireland and they are probably rising at a rate of over 10,000 per year.

Diet and physical activity

A balance of food intake and physical activity is necessary for a healthy weight. The foods we individually consume and our participation in physical activity are the result of a complex supply and production system. The growing research evidence that energy dense foods promote obesity is impressive and convincing. These are the foods that are high in fat, sugar and starch. Of these potentially the most significant promoter of weight gain is fat and foods from the top shelf of the food pyramid including spreads (butter and margarine), cakes and biscuits, and confectionery, when combined are the greatest contributors to fat intake in the Irish diet (see figure 2.2, page 32).

In company with their adult counterparts Irish children are also consuming large amounts of energy dense foods outside the home. A recent survey revealed that slightly over half of these children ate sweets at least once a day and roughly a third of them had fizzy drinks and crisps with the same regularity. Sugar sweetened carbonated drinks are thought to contribute to obesity and for this reason the World Health Organisation has expressed serious concerns at the high and increasing consumption of these drinks by children.

Physical activity is an important determinant of body weight. Over recent decades there has been a marked decline in demanding physical work and this has been accompanied by more sedentary lifestyles generally and reduced leisure-time activity. These observable changes, which are supported by data from most European countries and the United States, suggest that physical inactivity has made a significant impact on the increase in overweight and obesity being seen today.

It is now widely accepted that adults shoud be involved in 45-60 minutes, and children should be involved in at least 60 minutes per day of moderate physical activity in order to prevent excess weight gain.

The cost to society

Being overweight today not only signals increased risk of medical problems but also exposes people to serious psychosocial problems due mainly to widespread prejudice against fat people. Prejudice against obese people seems to border on the socially acceptable in Ireland. It crops up consistently in surveys covering groups such as employers, teachers, medical and healthcare personnel, and the media. It occurs among adolescents and children, even very young children.

Because obesity is associated with premature death, excessive morbidity and serious psychosocial problems the damage it causes to the welfare of citizens is extremely serious and for this reason government intervention is necessary and warranted. In economic terms, a figure of approximately €30million has been estimated for in-patient costs alone in 2003 for a number of Irish hospitals. This year about 2,000 premature deaths in Ireland will be attributed to obesity and the numbers are growing relentlessly. Diseases which proportionally more obese people suffer from than the general population include hypertension, type 2 diabetes, angina, heart attack and osteoarthritis. There are indirect costs also such as days lost to the workplace due to illness arising from obesity and output foregone as a result of premature death. Using the accepted EU environmental cost benefit method, these deaths alone may be costing the state as much as €4bn per year.

The challenge for society

The social determinants of physical activity include factors such as socio-economic status, education level, gender, family and peer group influences as well as individual perceptions of the benefits of physical activity. The environmental determinants include geographic location, time of year, and proximity of facilities such as open spaces, parks and safe recreational areas generally. The environmental factors have not yet been as well studied as the social ones and this research gap needs to be addressed. Clearly there is a public health imperative to ensure that relevant environmental policies maximise opportunities for active transport, recreational physical activity and total physical activity.

It is clear that concerted policy initiatives must be put in place if the predominantly negative findings of research regarding the determinants of food consumption and physical activity are to be accepted, and they must surely be accepted by government if the rapid increase in the incidence of obesity with all its negative consequences for citizens is to be reversed. So far actions surrounding nutrition policies have concentrated mostly on actions that are within the remit of the Department of Health and Children such as implementing the dietary guidelines. These are important but government must now look at the totality of policies that influence the type and supply of food that its citizens eat and the range and quality of opportunities that are available to citizens to engage in physical activity. This implies a fundamental examination of existing agricultural, industrial, economic and other policies and a determination to change them if they do not enable people to eat healthily and partake in physical activity.

The current crisis in obesity prevalence requires a population health approach for adults and children in addition to effective weight-reduction management for individuals who are severely overweight. This entails addressing the obesogenic environment where people live, creating conditions over time which lead to healthier eating and more active living, and protecting people from the widespread availability of unhealthy food and beverage options in addition to sedentary activities that take up all of their leisure time.

The way forward

People of course have a fundamental right to choose to eat what they want and to be as active as they wish. That is not the issue. What the National Taskforce on Obesity has had to take account of is that many forces are actively impeding change for those well aware of the potential health and well-being consequences to themselves of overweight and obesity. The

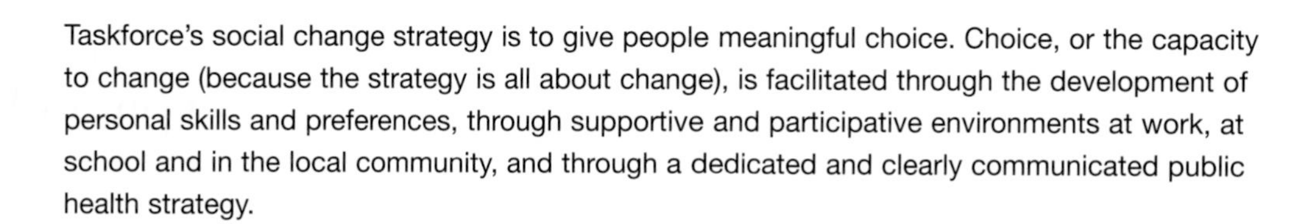

Taskforce's social change strategy is to give people meaningful choice. Choice, or the capacity to change (because the strategy is all about change), is facilitated through the development of personal skills and preferences, through supportive and participative environments at work, at school and in the local community, and through a dedicated and clearly communicated public health strategy.

What can the government do in the face of the growing epidemic of obesity?

High-level cabinet support will be necessary to implement the Taskforce's recommendations. The approach to implementation must be characterised by joined-up thinking, real practical engagement by the public and private sectors, the avoidance of duplication of effort or cross-purpose approaches, and the harnessing of existing strategies and agencies. The range of government departments with roles to play is considerable. The Taskforce outlines the different contributions that each relevant department can make in driving its strategy forward. It also emphasises its requirement that all phases of the national strategy for healthy eating and physical activity are closely monitored, analysed and evaluated.

The vision of the Taskforce is expressed as: ***An Irish society that enables people through health promotion, prevention and care to achieve and maintain healthy eating and active living throughout their lifespan.***

Its high-level goals are expressed as follows:

- The Taoiseach's Office will ensure that an integrated, consistent and proactive approach will be taken across all government departments, agencies and public bodies in addressing the problem of overweight/obesity.

- The private sector has an important role; it acknowledges it has a responsibility and will be proactive in addressing the issue of overweight/obesity.

- The public sector, the private sector and the community and voluntary sectors should work in partnership to promote healthy eating and active living to address overweight/obesity.

- Individuals should be personally empowered to tackle overweight/obesity and sensitive interventions should be developed to support them.

Its recommendations, over eighty in all, relate to actions across six broad sectors: high-level government; education; social and community; health; food, commodities, production and supply; and the physical environment.

In developing its recommendations the Taskforce have taken account of the complex, multi-sectoral and multi-faceted determinants of diet and physical activity. This strategy poses challenges for government, within individual departments, inter-departmentally and in developing partnerships with the commercial sector. Equally it challenges the commercial sector to work in partnership with government. The framework required for such initiative has at its core the rights and benefits of the individual. Health promotion is fundamentally about empowerment, whether at the individual, the community or the policy level.

Background

BACKGROUND

The environment in which people live should make healthy eating and active living the easier choice. However it is recognised that throughout life, from growth in the womb, through childhood, into adulthood and onwards, people are exposed to a range of influences that can increase their risk of becoming overweight and obese. Overweight and obesity pose a global health challenge. In 2000 the World Health Organisation (WHO) highlighted the problem of increasing global prevalence of obesity. In 2002 the Danish Presidency of the EU recognised that obesity was a major cause of a range of serious diseases, including cardiovascular disease, type 2 diabetes and hypertension. To facilitate European action, Denmark organised an international conference on obesity, to which all member states were invited. The EU resolutions from this meeting recommended that the Commission would:

- support member states in their efforts to address the issue of obesity immediately, especially obesity in children, by developing innovative measures and approaches concerning nutrition and physical activity
- strengthen research on obesity (while the member states simultaneously carry out action on obesity based on current scientific evidence including the establishment of national obesity taskforces)
- ensure that the prevention of obesity is taken into account in all relevant Community policies, and in particular in the framework of the programme of community action in the field of public health.

Addressing obesity is a priority of the EU's Public Health Action Programme for 2003-2008. The programme is funding a five-year EU-wide Nutrition and Physical Activity network to facilitate collaboration on obesity prevention strategies.

In March 2004 the Minister for Health and Children, Micheál Martin TD, established the National Taskforce on Obesity (NTFO).

The terms of reference of the Taskforce

Having regard to current national polices, in particular the Cardiovascular Health Strategy[1] and the Health Promotion Strategy 2000 to 2005[2], to develop a strategy to halt the rise and reverse the prevalence of obesity including:

- the current rates and trends of obesity in Ireland
- the determinants of obesity in Irish society
- the current and future impact on the health services and society as a whole from the growing trend in obesity
- best practice in the prevention, detection and treatment of obesity
- how best to create the social and physical environments that make it easier for children and adults to eat more healthily and be more active on a regular basis.

Present a strategy document to the Minister for Health and Children.

Infrastructure

The investment by the government in recent years, especially in support of the implementation of the Cardiovascular Health Strategy, Building Healthier Hearts[1], has put much of the infrastructure in place to address overweight and obesity prevention. This includes the appointment, for the first time, of physical activity co-ordinators by each health board and the introduction of twenty-six additional community dietitians.

This government has been proactive in relation to overweight and obesity and has responded through many programmes and initiatives, such as:

- Nutrition Health Promotion Framework for Action[3]
- Recommendations for a Food and Nutrition Policy (Nutrition Advisory Group, 1995)[4]
- Twelve-year National Healthy Eating Campaign
- National Physical Activity Campaign
- National Play Policy for Children
- National Obesity Campaign 2004 (following establishment of the Taskforce).

Intersectoral working

The report of the Cardiovascular Health Strategy Group, Building Healthier Hearts, was launched by An Taoiseach in July 1999 and sets out the blueprint for tackling heart disease in Ireland in the long term. The successful implementation of the Cardiovascular Health Strategy is the result of a number of factors including the government commitment to implementing the broad-ranging multisectoral recommendations in the Strategy.

Obesity, like heart disease, is associated with social, economic and biological determinants which include:

- the physical environment
- working conditions
- income and social status
- educational attainment
- ethnicity
- biological and genetic make-up
- healthy child development
- personal health practices and skills
- social support networks.

Several of these determinants fall outside the reach of the health sector, which demonstrates that if the issue of obesity is to be successfully addressed, there is a need for cross-sectoral co-operation between government departments[5,6].

Strategic framework

The NTFO recommendations have been informed by national strategies and policies, by EU initiatives and by WHO strategies, which Ireland has endorsed. As with the national health strategy Quality and Fairness[7] the principles of equity, people-centeredness, quality and accountability are inherent in the NTFO recommendations. The Health Promotion Strategy[2], the Cardiovascular Health Strategy[1], the National Play Policy[8], the school syllabi for physical education, Social, Personal and Health Education (SPHE), Biology and Home Economics as well as the Breastfeeding Policy[9] have direct relationships with the NTFO's objective. The NTFO supports and endorses the recommendations of these strategies and policy documents and presses for the implementation of their recommendations. In addition, as a member of the World Health Organisation, Ireland has signed up to strategies and policies that have a direct impact on the prevention and treatment of overweight and obesity. The Ottawa Charter[10] and the Jakarta Declaration[11] are the bases of health promotion principles endorsed by the Health Promotion Strategy. Ireland recently signed up to the WHO Global Strategy on Diet, Physical Activity and Health[12], which has made recommendations in relation to the responsibility of WHO, Ireland and the public and private sector in the area of diet, physical activity, and health. All these strategies and policies have informed the principles underlying the recommendations of the NTFO.

THE CONSULTATION PROCESS

Sub-Committees (see appendix A for membership)

Three ad hoc sub-committees were established as follows:

- Private Sector Sub-committee
- Public Sector Sub-committee
- Treatment and Detection Sub-committee.

The work undertaken by the sub-committees included:

- agreeing key stakeholders to be invited to make submissions
- discussing the main issues arising from submissions and deciding how to address them
- drafting recommendations
- reporting back to the plenary group.

Consultation process

The Taskforce carried out a comprehensive and systematic consultation process.

- Key stakeholders were invited to make submissions to the Taskforce (as identified by sub-committees).
- An advertisement was placed in the national press inviting all interested members of the public, organisations and groups to make submissions to the Taskforce.
- Over 300 submissions were received from individuals, the public and private sectors, and other groups and organisations (individuals: 104, organisations: 199). The submissions were collated by the National Nutrition Surveillance Centre and circulated to Taskforce members.
- The Taskforce is aware of the needs, opinions and feelings of those who are currently overweight/obese. Submissions were received from people, individually or as represented by groups, who were both overweight and obese and from organisations who support people in managing their weight. It was not possible, in the given timeframe, to comprehensively consult with people who are presently overweight/obese (see recommendations in Chapter 5).
- Sub-committees invited further formal submissions from some of those who made initial submissions. The sub-committees also in some instances requested a meeting with some of the stakeholders to provide further information as appropriate.
- Everyone who made a submission was invited to a consultation day held on 3 September in Dublin City University where attendance was in excess of 200. This consultation day was facilitated by Halley and Associates. Two reports were produced subsequently by Halley and Associates and were circulated to all who attended.

The Taskforce is mindful of the government commitment in the National Children's Strategy to consult with children and young people on matters which affect them and is conscious of the need to engage with children and young people on the issues of obesity and overweight. However, consultation with children and young people, if it is to be meaningful, should be structured and comprehensive and the timescale available to the Taskforce to complete its strategy and report to the Minister for Health and Children did not allow for such a structured and comprehensive process. The Taskforce had no wish to carry out a tokenistic consultation and took the view that while consultation should take place, there was not sufficient time in the present instance to perform the task adequately. The Taskforce believes that the views of children and young people should be sought in relation to its recommendations and in furthering the implementation of these (see recommendations in Chapter 5).

Obesity conference

A conference entitled 'Tackling Obesity Together – Every Step Counts' was convened by the Health Promotion Unit of the Department of Health and Children, Republic of Ireland, and the Health Promotion Agency for Northern Ireland on 25- 26 November 2004 in the Slieve Russell Hotel, Cavan.

This conference aimed to:

- help address the prevention and management of overweight and obesity by focusing specifically on the theme of integrating physical activity and good nutrition
- reach agreement on strategic approaches which will facilitate the development of a consistent, integrated approach to preventing and tackling obesity, involving all stakeholders and interest groups
- provide a further focus for the respective Taskforces on Obesity
- help inform emerging policies and practice at national and local level.

Plenary meetings

Eleven plenary meetings were held by the Taskforce, including a two-day meeting facilitated by Halley and Associates. At this meeting an outline template, which was used to frame the Strategy, was agreed by the Taskforce and the vision, high-level goals and draft recommendations were developed. Informative presentations were made to the Taskforce on a range of subject matters (see appendix B).

Drafting the strategy

The secretariat, in consultation with the Taskforce, gathered evidence to inform the national goals and recommendations made by the Taskforce. This information along with the consultation day reports, the summary of collated submissions, key messages and outcomes from the obesity conference, and the collation of international data describing the determinants and prevalence of obesity were used to inform the drafting of the Strategy.

1 The extent of OVERWEIGHT and OBESITY

KEY POINTS

- Overweight/Obesity is measured in adults by Body Mass Index (BMI). Overweight = BMI ≥ 25.0 kg/m^2; Obese = BMI ≥ 30.0 kg/m^2.
- Rates of obesity are growing worldwide. In the last ten years the level of obesity in Europe has grown by at least 10% and up to 50% in some countries.
- In Ireland, obesity in adults is increasing by at least 1% every year.
- Obesity tends to be higher in men, those aged over 35, those with no/some education and those in lower socio-economic groups.
- Classification of children as overweight or obese is more difficult than for adults because height, weight, age and gender need to be considered.
- Levels of overweight and obesity in Irish adolescent girls (aged 13 and 15) are higher than the international average.
- Despite different ways of measuring obesity in children, all methods show that obesity in children is increasing.

1 The extent of OVERWEIGHT and OBESITY

Definition of obesity

While there is some debate as to whether obesity should be classified as a disease rather than a predisposing condition[13], an expert consultation on obesity convened by the World Health Organisation defined obesity as a disease in which excess body fat has accumulated to an extent that health is adversely affected[14].

The World Health Organisation has used Body Mass Index (BMI) to estimate the prevalence and associated risks of overweight and obesity within a population[14]. The BMI is calculated as:

$$\text{BMI} = \frac{\text{Weight (kg)}}{\text{Height squared (m}^2\text{)}}$$

Studies have shown that BMI is significantly correlated with total body fat content for the majority of individuals[15]. The classification of overweight and obesity, according to BMI, is shown in Table 1.1.

Table 1.1: Classification of overweight and obesity in adults according to BMI

Classification	BMI (kg/m²)	Risk of co morbidities
Underweight	<18.5	Low (but risk of other clinical problems increased)
Normal range	18.5-24.9	Average
Overweight	≥25.0	
Pre-obese	25.0-29.9	Increased
Obese class I	30.0-34.9	Moderate
Obese class II	35.0-39.9	Severe
Obese class III	≥40.0	Very severe

While BMI is a convenient measurement for a general population it may not be appropriate for certain individuals. BMI does not distinguish weight associated with fat from weight associated with water or muscle; therefore athletes may have a high BMI but very little percentage body fat. BMI also gives no indication of body fat distribution. This is important because it is not just the amount or the composition of excess weight that affects health, but also where the fat is stored in the body. Obese individuals with excess fat deposited around the abdomen ('apple-shaped') are more likely than those who have fat deposited on the hips and buttocks ('pear-shaped') to develop health problems. A measurement of waist to hip ratio (WHR) is an appropriate method of identifying patients with abdominal fat accumulation. The waist is measured at the narrowest point and the hips are measured at the widest point. A high WHR is defined as >1.0 in men and >0.85 in women. WHO recommends the use of waist circumference measurement because it correlates closely with BMI and WHR, and is an approximate index of intra-abdominal fat mass and total body fat.

Changes in waist circumference indicate changes in risk factors for cardiovascular and other chronic diseases. There is an increased risk of metabolic complications for (Caucasian) men with a waist circumference ≥102cm, and women with a waist circumference ≥88cm.

Self-perception of body size

There is a common perception that 'obesity' is a highly visible state of overweight. In fact, the BMI cut-off for obesity is quite low. Adults are poor at identifying overweight in themselves, while the levels of overweight and obesity in Ireland demonstrate that a substantial proportion of our adult population is currently overweight or obese. The IUNA study found that people who claimed that their weight was fine for their age were more likely to have higher BMIs[16]. Younger people (18-35) were most likely to think that their weight was fine for their age, as were unskilled workers, students and those with normal weight[16]. In older adults, 27% of those aged 51 to 64 years were obese and 44% were overweight but 50% of this group thought their weight was fine for their age.

In a recent UK study only 25% of parents recognised overweight in their child. Among overweight parents, 27% of mothers and 61% of fathers were unconcerned about their weight[17]. Acknowledgment of excess weight and an understanding of its health consequences are essential first steps in tackling obesity.

A global problem

The prevalence of overweight and obesity has increased rapidly over the past two decades and it has been described by WHO as 'a global epidemic'. While originally obesity was associated with developed, western societies, now low-income countries are experiencing an obesity epidemic. In 1995 there was an estimated 200 million obese adults globally. In 2000 more than 300 million adults were estimated to be obese: 132 million in developed countries and 170 million in other countries[18].

Certain countries have experienced a staggering increase in obesity rates over the last three decades as indicated in Figure 1.1. The World Health Organisation estimates that the growth in the number of severely overweight adults is to double that of underweight adults during the period 1995-2025[14]. Crude projections, extrapolating existing data, suggest that by the year 2025 levels of obesity could be as high as 45-50% in the USA, between 30-40% in Australia, England and Mauritius and over 20% in Brazil[19].

Figure 1.1: The growing epidemic of obesity

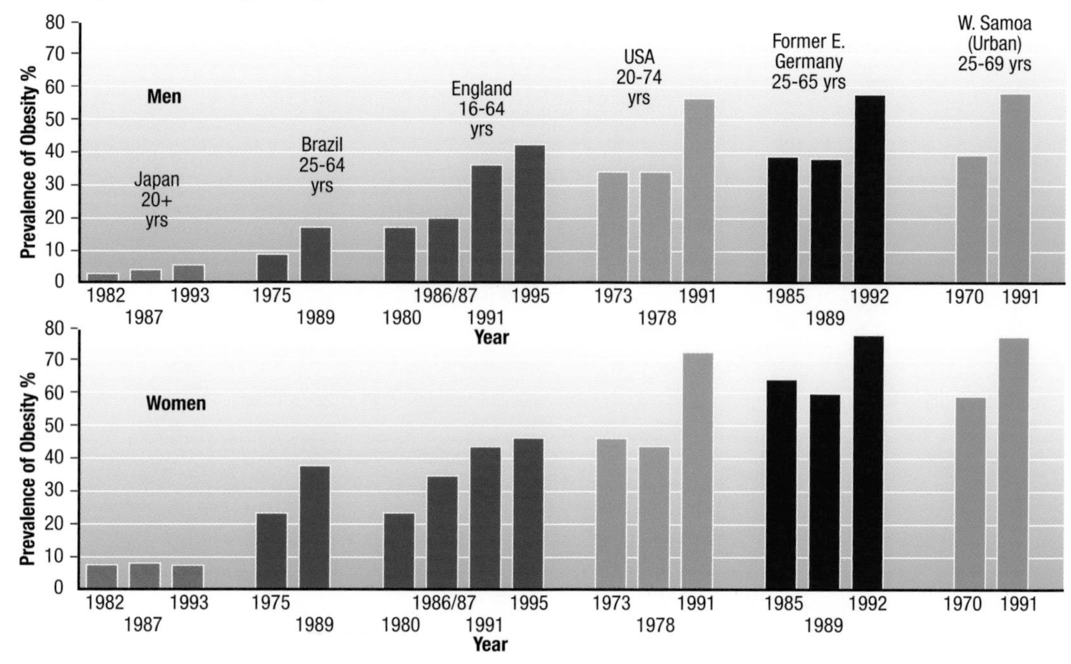

(Source: IOTF, 2002)

Adult mean BMI levels of 22-23 kg/m^2 are found in Africa and Asia, while levels of 25-27 kg/m^2 are prevalent across Europe, and in some Latin American, North African and Pacific Island countries[19]. Current obesity levels range from below 5% in China, Japan and certain African nations to over 75% in urban Samoa[19]. Data from the United States show that the prevalence of overweight and obesity among adults 20–74 years of age increased from 47% during 1976–80 to 65 % during 1999–2002. During this period the prevalence of obesity among adults 20–74 years of age increased from 15% to 31 %[20].

In many developing countries undergoing economic changes, rising levels of obesity often coexist in the same population with chronic undernutrition. In low-income countries, obesity is more common in middle-aged women, people of higher socio-economic status and those living in urban communities. In more affluent countries, obesity is not only common in the middle-aged, but is becoming increasingly prevalent among younger adults and children. In these countries obesity is associated with lower socio-economic status, especially among women, and is as prevalent in rural as urban populations[14].

Europe

Obesity is a major public health problem throughout Europe. Current data from individual national studies suggest that in European countries between 10% and 20% of men and 10% and 25% of women are obese [21] (Figure 1.2).

Rates of obesity vary between different countries, but the prevalence of obesity in most European countries has increased by 10-50% in the last ten years. The most dramatic increase has been in the UK where prevalence has almost tripled in twenty years. UK figures for 2002 showed that 22% of men and 23.5% of women were obese and that almost 66% of men and 50% of women had a BMI ≥25 kg/m^2 (Figure 1.2a & b) – almost 24 million adults[22]. A survey in Northern Ireland reported that 39% of adults were overweight and 19% were obese; 20% of women were obese compared to 17% of men[23]. Rates of obesity in the Baltic Republics are among the highest in the world[24].

Figure 1.2: Prevalence of adult obesity in Europe BMI ≥ 30 kg/m^2

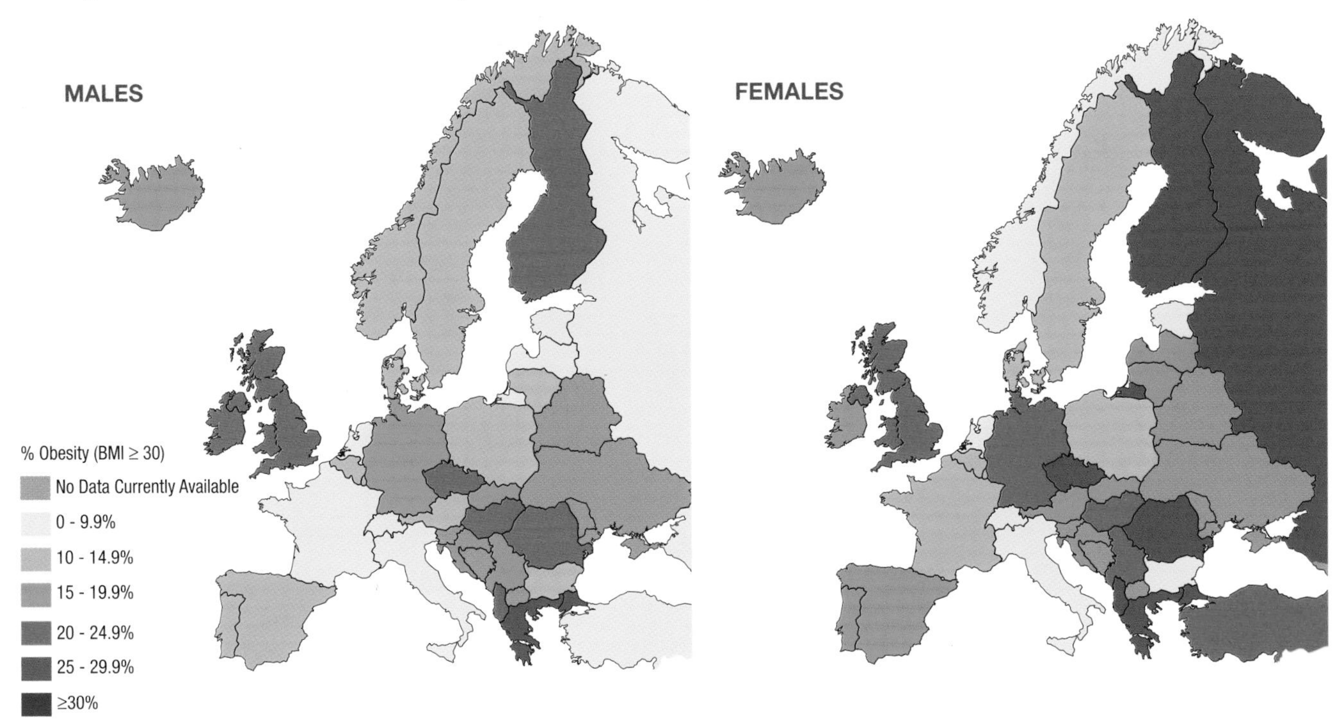

(Source, IOTF, 2003)

Figure 1.2a: Estimated EU country prevalence of overweight and obesity

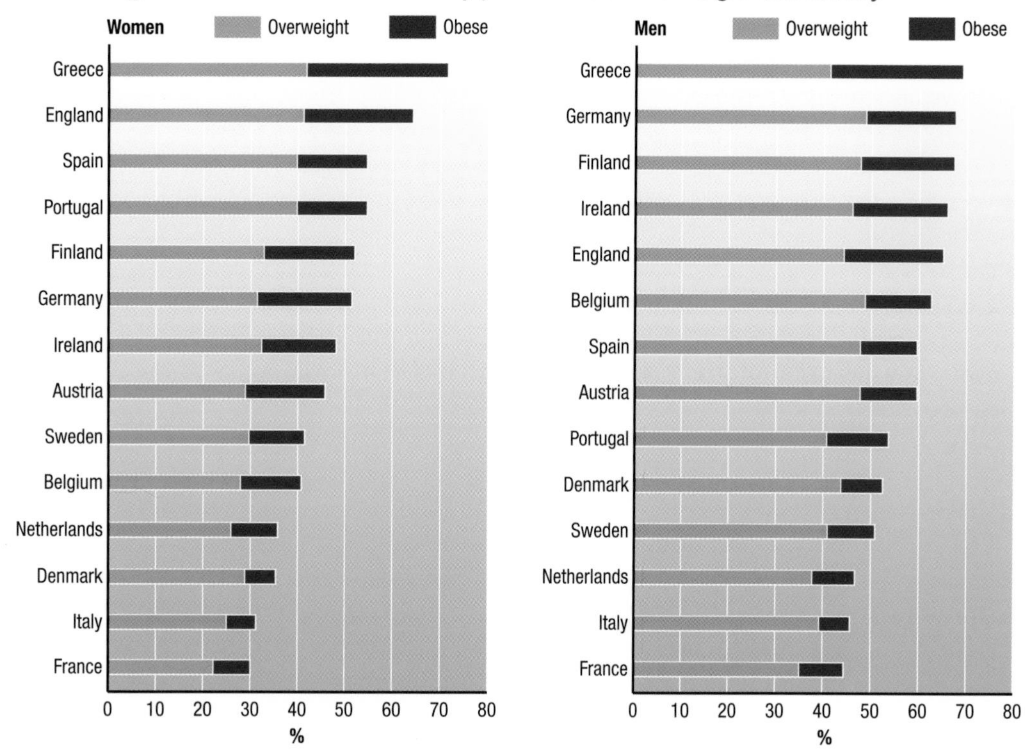

*Restricted Age Group
**Germany overweight figures derived from WHO MONICA studies

Figure 1.2b: EU Accession Countries

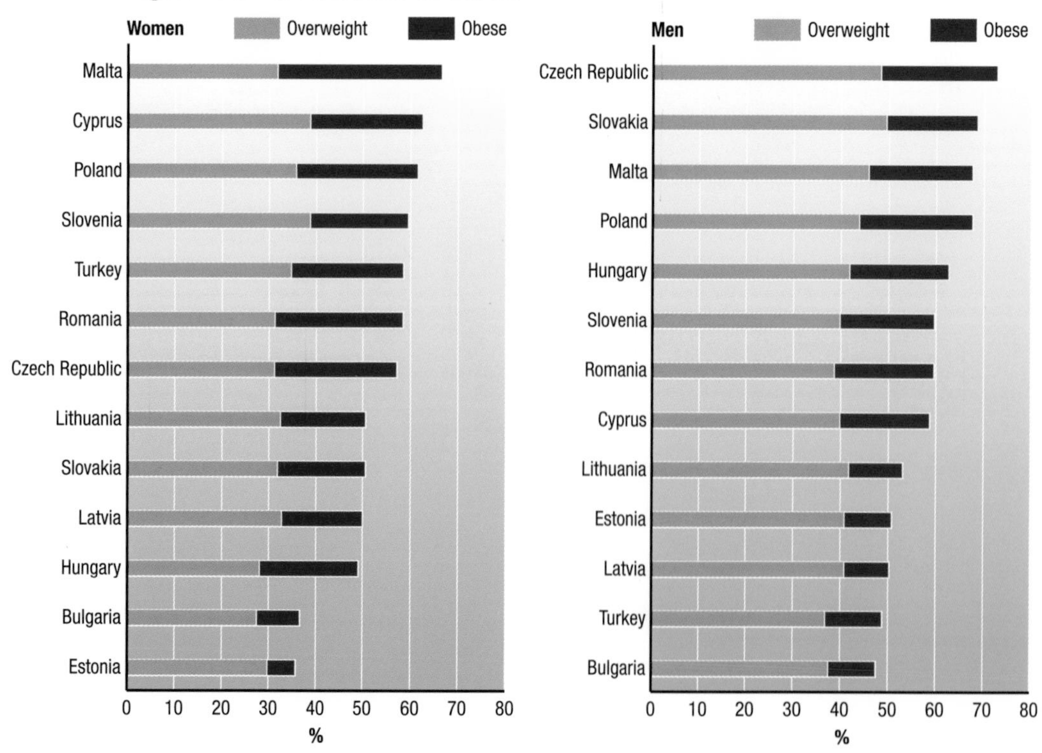

(Source: IOTF, 2002)

Obesity in Ireland

Obesity prevalence in Ireland has been estimated using two different methods:

- Direct measurement of weight and heights of a population sample (the 1990 Irish National Nutrition Survey[26] and the North/South Ireland Food Consumption Survey, 2001[16], n=1,379)
- Self-reported weights and heights (SLÁN, 1998[27], n=6,539; SLÁN, 2002[28], n=5,992).

Both methods have advantages in estimating the epidemic problem and provide us with important trend information. Direct measurements give a more reliable estimation of individual weights and heights. However this method is often not feasible in large-scale population surveys. Self-reported measurements are prone to underestimation of weight and overestimation of heights but have the advantage that trends over time and across social groups can be undertaken. Hayes et al (2004) recently examined the agreement between self-reported and clinical classifications of obesity in the SLÁN surveys. As expected, overweight and obese respondents were more likely to under-report but when this effect is corrected for, the estimates of obesity tally closely with the direct-measured data[29].

The North/South Ireland Food Consumption survey indicates that 39% of the adult population were overweight and 18% were obese[16]. A higher percentage of men were overweight and obese compared to women[16].

A number of factors have been linked to obesity, including age, gender and socio-economic status. In developed countries the natural pattern is an increase in body weight with ageing, at least up to 50-60 years old (in both men and women). This trend can be seen in the Irish population (Figure 1.3)[16]. The decline in prevalence after this peak is thought to be partly attributed to the lower survival rate of obese individuals. Clear gender differences are seen in most countries with more women than men being obese; however the prevalence of obesity in men has increased so rapidly in Ireland that it now exceeds the prevalence of obesity in women[16, 30].

Figure 1.3: Age and gender distribution of obesity, 1990 and 2000

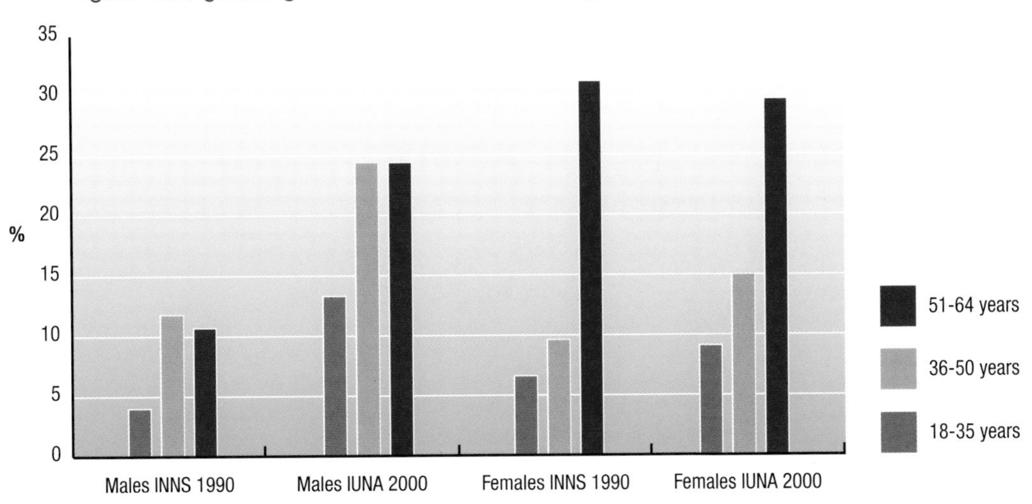

(Source: IUNA, 2001)

According to the SLÁN data, rates in Irish adults have risen from 11.3% of men in 1998 to 14.4% in 2002 and from 9.3% of women in 1998 to 11.8% in 2002[28] (Figure 1.4) which indicates a minimum 1% increase in obesity per annum. The prevalence of adults who are overweight has also increased significantly from 39.6% in men in 1998 to 41.9% in 2002 and from 24.9% of women in 1998 to 26.5% in 2002.

Figure 1.4 : Gender distribution of obesity in 1998 and 2002

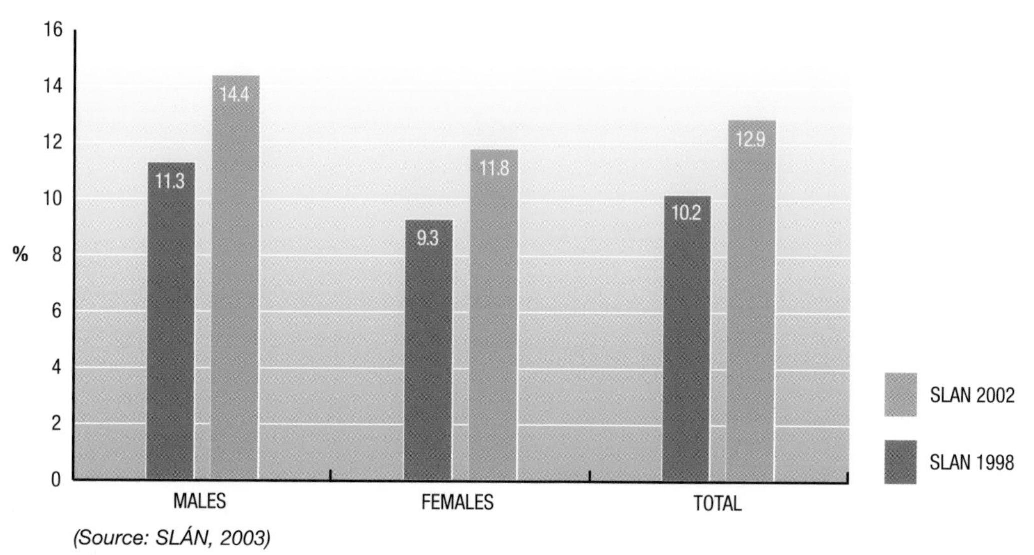

(Source: SLÁN, 2003)

In Ireland educational level is a strong predictor of health outcome. Those with lower levels of education were more likely to be obese[16,30]. Those who have some education have higher levels of obesity than those who have completed secondary or tertiary education. However, the rates of obesity have increased across all educational levels since 1998[28] (Figure 1.5).

Figure 1.5: Distribution of obesity among different educational groups

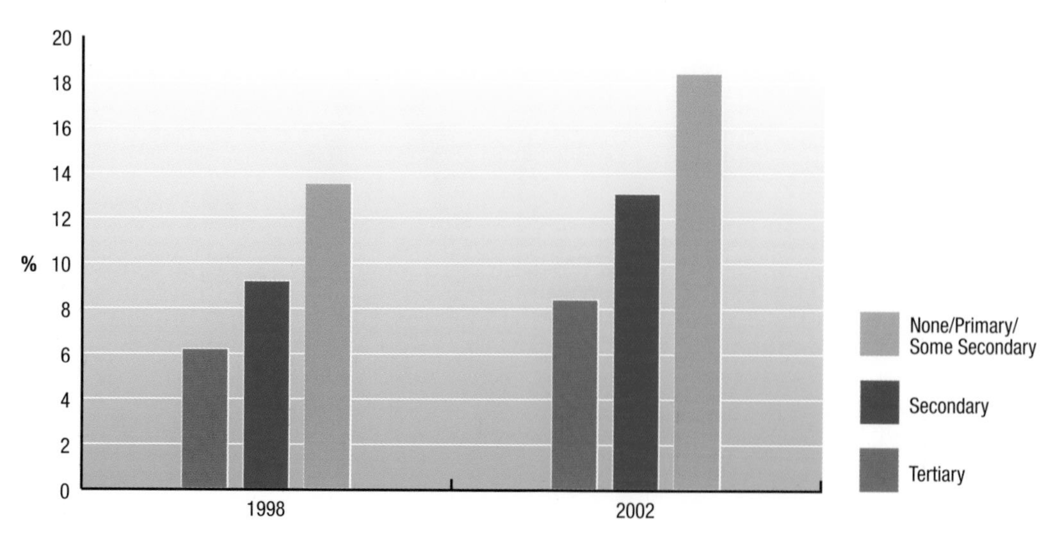

(Source: SLÁN, 2003)

Patterns have also emerged across socio-economic groups. In developed countries, such as Ireland, levels of obesity are higher in the lower socio-economic groups (5 and 6) (Figure 1.6) [28]. In developing countries this relationship is reversed. While obesity levels have increased across all socio-economic groupings the increases are most notable in the lower social classes 5 and 6[28].

Figure 1.6: Distribution of obesity among different social groups

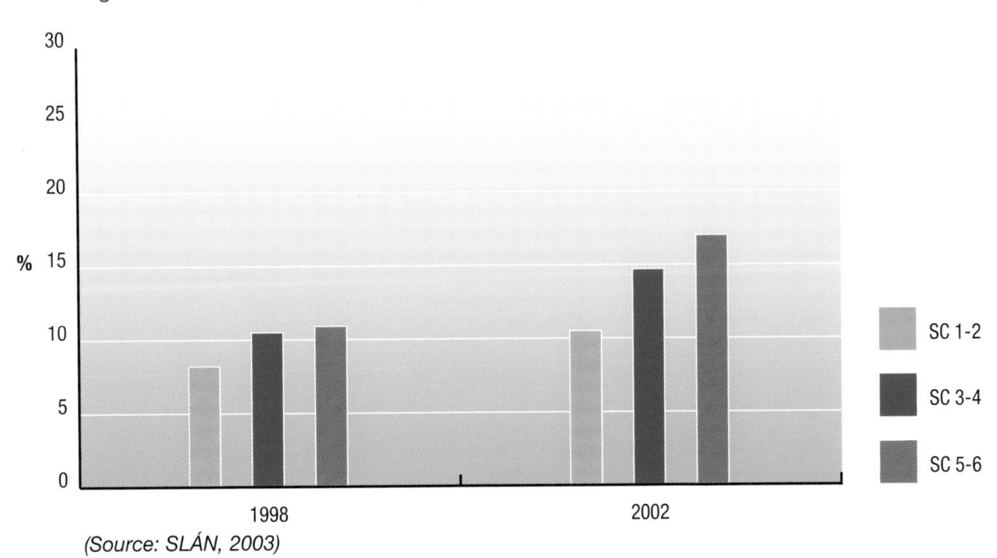

(Source: SLÁN, 2003)

Internationally the transition from a rural to an urban lifestyle is associated with increased levels of obesity, which has been linked with dramatic changes in lifestyles (for example increased consumption of high energy dense foods and decreased physical activity). However, while levels of obesity have increased in both rural and urban areas in Ireland there is little or no difference in levels of obesity between those living in rural or urban areas (Figure 1.7) [28].

Figure 1.7: Distribution of obesity in urban and rural areas

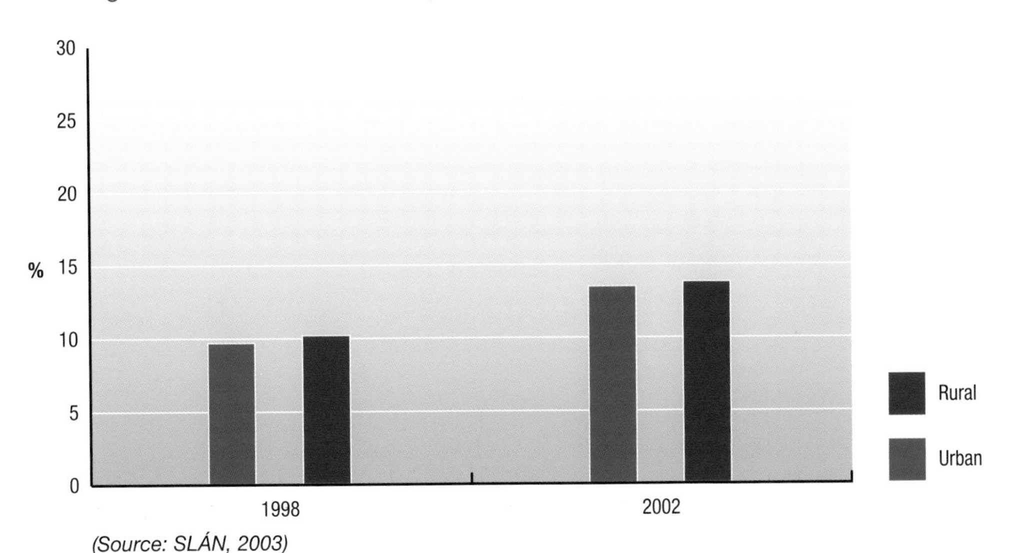

(Source: SLÁN, 2003)

OBESITY IN CHILDHOOD

Assessing obesity in children

It can be very difficult to distinguish children who are at risk of overweight from normal children[31]. Measurement of overweight/obesity in children is not straightforward because BMI in childhood changes substantially with age and is different between girls and boys.

- o Weight for height/length measurements are a common means of assessing populations of children, particularly children under five years, and are used to classify both undernutrition and overnutrition [32].
- o Body Mass Index

  Estimations of BMI values in children and adolescents depend on comparisons with population reference data, using cut-off points in the BMI for age and gender distribution (BMI percentiles). However, a variety of cut-offs and reference data is currently in use:
  - 1990 UK reference data for age and sex[33]: obese children are those with a BMI>98th centile and overweight children are those with a BMI >91st centile
  - The majority of international literature uses a definition of BMI >85th centile of reference data for at-risk of overweight and BMI >95th centile of reference data for overweight. In the United States, the 85th and 95th centiles of BMI for age and sex, based on a nationally representative survey, have been recommended[31]
  - The International Obesity Taskforce (IOTF) proposed that the adult cut-off points (25 and 30 kg/m^2) be linked to BMI for age centiles for girls and boys to provide child cut-off points[34].

Global childhood obesity

Childhood obesity is already epidemic in some areas and on the rise in others. Using existing WHO standards, data from 79 developing countries and a number of industrialised countries suggests that about 22 million children under five years are overweight worldwide[14].

The prevalence of overweight is, in general, higher among boys than girls, with the exception of the United States (See Table 1.2) [35]. In the United States in 1999 it was estimated that 13% of children aged 6-11 years and 14% of adolescents aged 12-19 years were overweight (overweight = age and sex specific BMI ≥ 95th percentile). Since the mid- 1970s the percentage of children who are overweight has nearly doubled (7% to 13%), and the percentage of adolescents who are overweight has almost tripled (from 5% to 14%)[36].

Table 1.2: Prevalence of overweight* children aged 6 to 8 years (%)

	USA 1988-91	China 1993	Russia 1994-95	South Africa 1994	Brazil 1989
Girls	24.2	12.2	17.8	20.3	10.5
Boys	21.3	14.1	25.6	25.0	12.8

Source: Popkin et al, 1996 (35)

*(*defined as BMI higher than the United States reference NHES 85th percentile)*

Europe

Excess body weight is now the most prevalent childhood disease in Europe, affecting one in six children. However, in some countries one in three children are overweight or obese (Figure 1.8) [23]. Type 2 diabetes and other weight-related diseases were, until recently, associated with middle age. They are now being increasingly observed in children.

Figure 1.8: Estimated prevalence of overweight and obesity in European children and adolescents

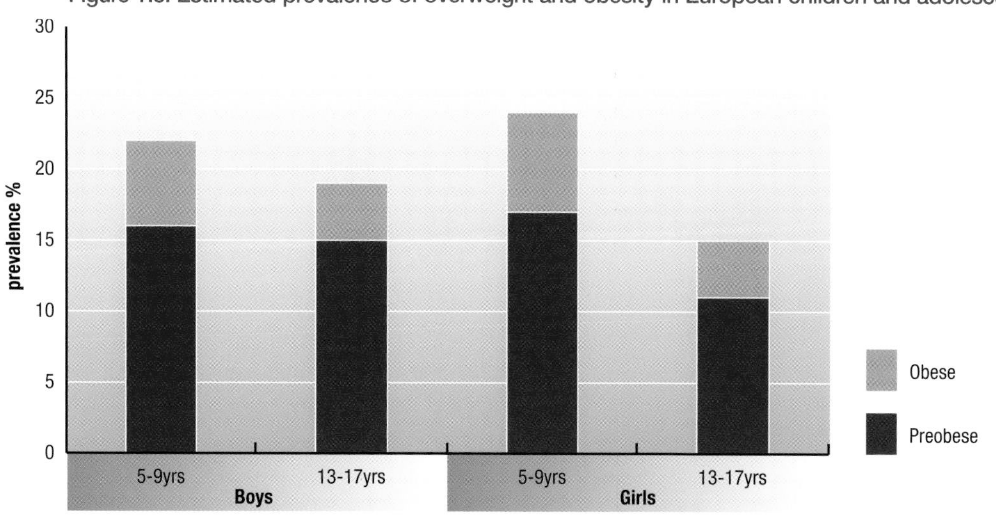

(Source: IOTF, 2003)

Using the IOTF-recommended cut-off criteria for overweight (which includes obesity) Lobstein and Frelut (2003) estimated the prevalence of childhood overweight and obesity in Europe using measured data from different surveys. Lower levels of overweight were found in children from central and eastern Europe[37]. The prevalence of overweight was found to be higher among the southern countries of Europe such as Greece and Italy[37]. The more developed countries surrounding the Mediterranean show prevalence rates for overweight children in the range 20-40%, while those in northern areas show rates in the range 10-20%[37]. The Health Survey for England (2002), using the IOTF classification, found that the prevalence of obesity in 2 to 15 year-olds was 5.5% for boys and 7.2% for girls [38]. In total a fifth of boys (21.8%) and over a quarter of girls (27.5%) were either overweight or obese [38].

Ireland

In Ireland, as in other countries, there is as yet a lack of consensus about assessment criteria for childhood obesity and currently no standards exist for assessing Irish children. This makes it difficult to estimate the true prevalence of obesity. Griffin et al (2004) found that in a study of inner city Dublin children the prevalence of overweight within the group differed between the four standard definitions of weight status (BMI for age [31,34,33] and actual relative weight[39].

In 1990 the Irish National Nutrition Survey reported that 1.9% of children aged 12-15 years were significantly overweight (BMI>26 kg/ m^2, which corresponds to a BMI>30 kg/ m^2 at full adult height) [26]. Using the same criterion to assess Dublin school children in 2000, Griffin et al (2004) found that the rate of significant overweight had trebled to 6%[39].

The Irish Oral Health Research Centre carried out the National Survey of Children's Dental Health 2001-02 and opportunistically included a weight and height measurement of each child[40]. These important results show that in Ireland levels of overweight (BMI for age and sex> 25 kg/m^2) and obesity (BMI for age and sex> 30 kg/m^2) in girls were the same or higher than in boys in all ages (see Figure 1.9 and Figure 1.10) [40]. Levels of overweight tended to decrease in girls in the older age groups but the younger aged girls (5 to 8) showed distinctly higher levels of overweight than the boys[40].

Figure 1.9: Percentage of children overweight (BMI for age and sex≥25kg/m^2)

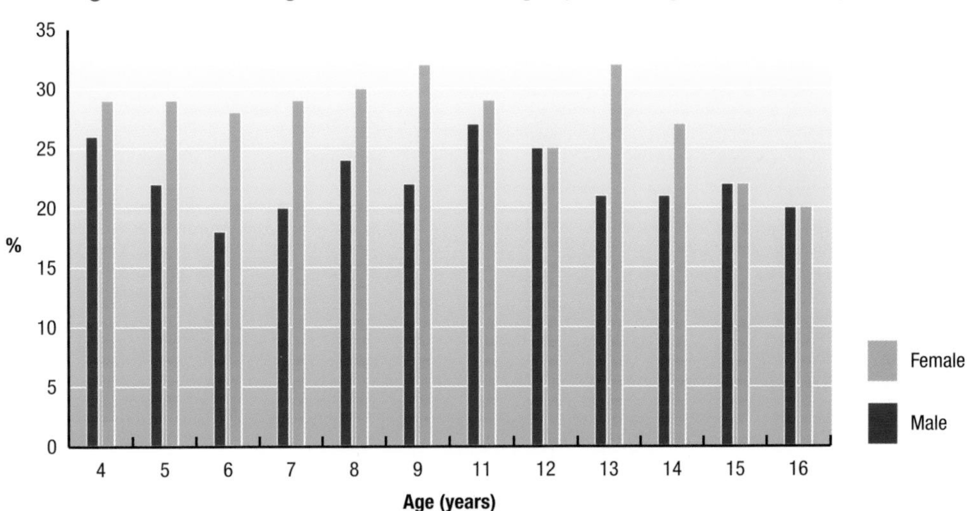

(Source: North South Survey of Height, Weight and Body Mass Index in Ireland, 2002)

Figure 1.10: Percentage of children obese (BMI for age and sex≥30kg/m^2)

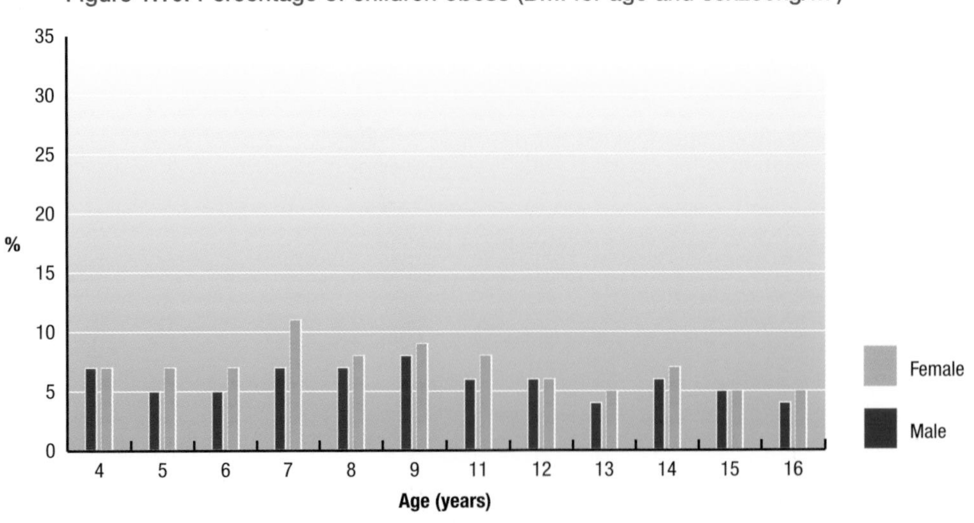

(Source: North South Survey of Height, Weight and Body Mass Index in Ireland, 2002)

The Health Behaviour in School-Aged Children (HBSC) study collected self-reported information on the height and weight of students in 2001-02 across twenty-nine countries worldwide. Age and gender-specific BMI international cut-off points were used to calculate the prevalence of overweight and obesity[34]. The children were then divided into overweight (pre-obese) and obese groups, which correspond to the adult BMI values of 25-29.9 and ≥ 30 kg/m^2 [41].

The study shows that there is a higher percentage of overweight (BMI for age and sex 25-29.9kg/m^2) 13- year-old boys than girls in Ireland while the reverse is true for 15- year-olds. The prevalence of overweight in boys was lower than international average in both ages but was higher in girls (Table 1.3)[41].

Irish 13-year-old boys reported higher levels of obesity (BMI for age and sex > 30 kg/m^2) than girls. However, the obesity levels in girls were slightly higher at age 15[41].
The prevalence of obesity in Ireland was lower than the international average in 15- year-old boys but higher in all 13-year-olds and 15-year-old girls (Table 1.3). Taken overall, rates for 13-year-olds were comparable with the international average in 13-year-olds but were lower than the international average for 15-year-old boys and higher for girls[41].

Table 1.3 The international average and Irish prevalence of overweight and obesity among 13 and 15 year olds

	13-year-olds		15-year-olds	
	Ireland 2002	HBSC 2002 average	Ireland 2002	HBSC 2002 average
Overweight boys	10.5	12	9.6	12.2
Obese boys	3.9	2.4	1.4	2.3
Total	**14.4**	**14.4**	**11.0**	**14.5**
Overweight girls	8.4	7.9	10.8	7.1
Obese girls	2.1	1.2	1.8	1.4
Total	**10.5**	**9.1**	**12.6**	**8.5**

(Source: WHO/HBSC, 2004 based on 2002 data)

The Health Behaviour in School Aged Children (HBSC) survey found that the percentage of young people dissatisfied with their body weight increased with age [41]. Approximately 20% of boys and girls aged eleven were dissatisfied with their body weight, which is lower than the HBSC international average of 28% for girls and 22% for boys of this age. Among 13-year-olds the HBSC average for body dissatisfaction was 37% for girls and 23% for boys[41]. Body dissatisfaction in Irish 13-year-old girls was higher than the average (40%) whereas the level in Irish 13-year-old boys was similar to the average. Among 15-year-olds, 48% of girls and 21% of boys were dissatisfied, which was higher than the HBSC averages of 42% and 20% respectively[41].

Adolescents may not be able to appropriately classify their body size in terms of weight and this can lead to a feeling of overweight rather than actual weight[41]. There are also clear gender differences in the manner in which girls and boys evaluate their bodies. This is evident in Figure 1.11 and Figure 1.12 when the measured BMI-for-age and sex (NSS)[40]are compared with self-reported BMI-for-age and sex (HBSC). Boys appear to underestimate their body size by approximately 30% (Figure 1.11) whereas girls greatly underestimate their size (Figure 1.12). Girls appear to feel greater cultural pressure to be 'slim' which leads to large discrepancies between what they perceive as being their 'right' size and their actual size.

Figure 1.11: Percentage of boys overweight and obese (BMI for age and sex $\geq$ 25 kg/m^2)

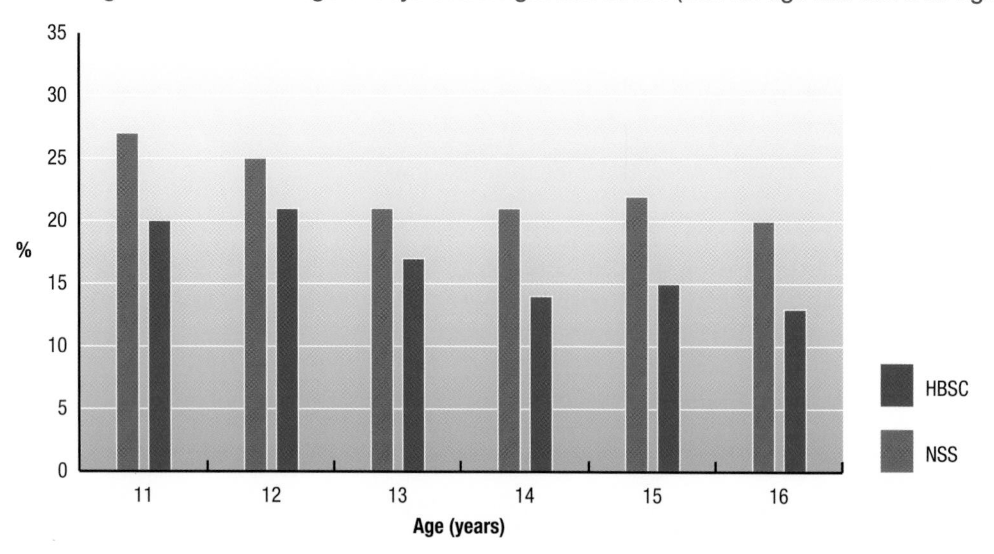

(Source: National Survey of Children's Dental Health 2001-02; HBSC 1998 and 2002)

Figure 1.12: Percentage of girls overweight and obese (BMI for age and sex $\geq$ 25 kg/m^2)

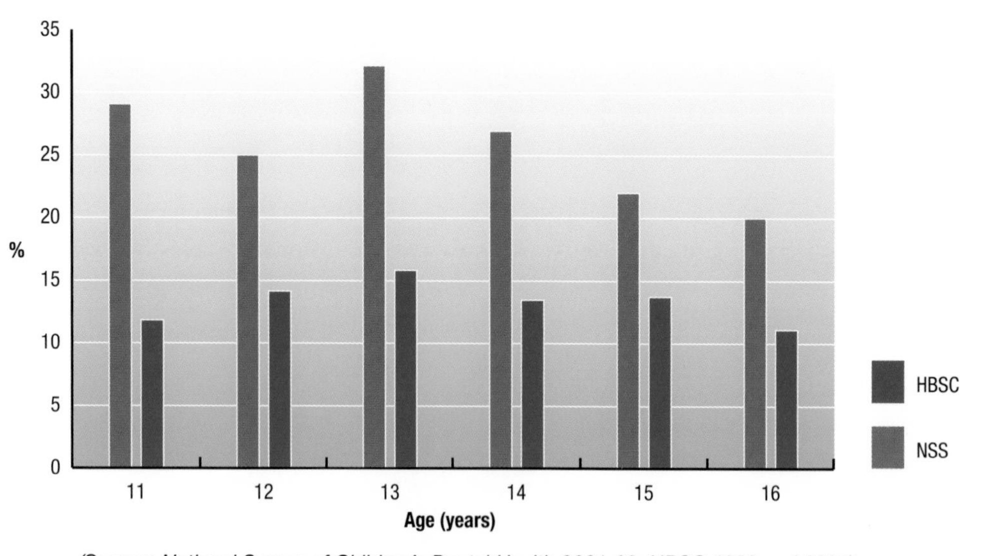

(Source: National Survey of Children's Dental Health 2001-02; HBSC 1998 and 2002)

While different definitional criteria and methodologies are used in different countries the trends for overweight and obesity are clearly upwards in young people from all sources.

2 DIET and PHYSICAL ACTIVITY Trends

KEY POINTS

- A high intake of energy dense foods and sugary drinks can lead to weight gain.
- High proportions of food prepared outside the home and large portion sizes may contribute to obesity.
- Regular physical activity protects against weight gain and obesity.
- Irish adults and children are not meeting physical activity recommendations.
- Adults require 45-60 minutes of moderate intensity activity to prevent the transition to overweight or obesity; 60-90 minutes per day for weight loss and the maintenance of weight loss.
- Children should be involved in at least 60 minutes of moderate physical activity each day.

Evidence of dietary factors contributing to obesity

There is convincing evidence that a high intake of energy dense foods promotes weight gain. Energy dense foods tend to be high in fat, sugars or starch[42]. Several studies have shown that high energy dense diets lead to 'passive over-consumption' of food. Humans have an innate ability to recognise foods with a high energy density and to appropriately down-regulate the bulk of food eaten in order to maintain energy balance[43]. Despite this ability, energy-dense diets can undermine the normal processes of appetite regulation in humans which causes an accidental positive energy balance that has consequently been termed 'passive over-consumption' [44].

The newly released dietary guidelines in the United States outline measures to reduce diet-related chronic disease, especially obesity, where dietary guidance is based on physical activity levels[45]. Given the critical importance of guidelines on healthy eating and active living in the light of the recommendations in this report, the development of new guidelines appropriate for Ireland remains a priority (see recommendations in Chapter 5).

Genes are important in determining a person's susceptibility to weight gain, but energy balance is determined by calorie intake and physical activity. Eating behaviours that have been linked to overweight and obesity include snacking/eating repeatedly, binge-eating patterns, and eating out, whereas breastfeeding has been shown to be protective against overweight and obesity. Candidate nutrient factors under investigation in the current literature include fat, carbohydrate type (including refined carbohydrates such as sugar), the glycaemic index† of foods and fibre[42].

Energy intake was shown to be positively associated with BMI in both men and women in the IUNA study[46]. People who consume fried food regularly and those who do not meet the recommendations from the bottom two shelves of the food pyramid (Fruit and Vegetables; Bread, Cereals and Potatoes) are more likely to be obese than those who consume fried food rarely and those who meet the food pyramid recommendations[28]. Those who meet the food pyramid recommendations from the Milk, Cheese and Yoghurt shelf are less likely to be obese. Restrained eating is also positively associated with BMI where individuals are aware of their weight and try to control their food intake[16].

† A measure of how quickly and how high specific foods raise blood sugar level

NUTRITION AND DIET

The Irish diet has changed dramatically over the last sixty years in terms of the variety of food available, food preference, and food technology. This is reflected in the comparison of the average daily nutrient intake today compared with that of 1948 (Table 2.1).

Table 2.1: Comparison of average Irish daily nutrient intake/capita/day

	Energy (MJ)	% Protein energy	% Fat energy	% Carbohydrate energy
*1948 National Nutrition Survey	13.04	13	29	58
*1990 Irish Nutrition and Dietetic Inst.	9.79	15	36	49
*1998 SLÁN	9.35	17	35	47
*2000 IUNA	9.3	16	35	44
*2002 SLÁN	9.04	18	33	50
WHO Recommendations		10-15	15-30	55-75

*(*Note different survey methodologies)*

Energy intakes

Energy intakes were higher overall in 1948 compared with 2002 and energy was mostly derived from carbohydrate sources. High levels of obesity and overweight were not observed in 1948. This can be partly explained by the greater levels of energy expenditure at that time owing to the fact that more people were in manual labour and motorised transport was not widely used. In 1948 daily nutrient intakes were within WHO recommendations[42]: these have not been met in recent years.

Energy intakes are generally higher in Irish males than females but they tend to decrease in both sexes with age. Actual energy intakes did not change significantly for the total population between 1998 and 2002. The reduction in energy intake from 1998 to 2002 was greater for women (49kcal/day) than for men (2kcal) [47].

The foods which contributed most to energy intake in the Irish diet, were meats (16%), breads (14%), potatoes (11%) and cakes and biscuits (9%) (Figure 2.1)[16].

Figure 2.1: Percentage contribution of food groups to energy intake

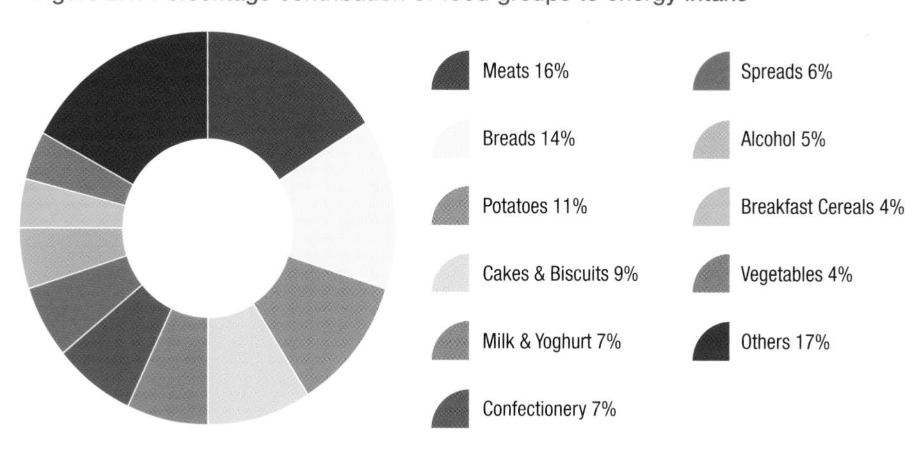

(Source: Irish Universities Nutrition Alliance, 2001)

Fat

Research evidence consistently shows that high-fat diets promote passive over-consumption of energy and increase of weight gain and obesity[48]. In the modern diet more energy is derived from fat and less is derived from carbohydrate. The energy density and fat content of food products and meals appear to have an important effect on the overall intake of food energy. Fat calories may be preferentially stored, while carbohydrate, alcohol and protein calories are expended more rapidly due to the body's limited capacity for storage [49].

The daily percentage of energy intake from fat has decreased by approximately 2% since 1998. This may be reflective of real changes in the Irish diet such as the shift towards low-fat dairy products. However it also may be as a result of people under-reporting foods that they know to be high in fat: studies have shown that foods high in fat and/or carbohydrates tend to be under-reported[50].

There is a strong age gradient with fat intake in males, with younger males obtaining greater amounts of energy from fat. Females aged between 18 to 34 and 35 to 54 tended to have similar intakes[28]. While intakes of saturated fats and monounsaturated fats (MUFAs) show a general trend of decreasing intake with age, intakes of polyunsaturated fats (PUFAs) tend to peak with men and women aged 35 to 54[47].

Reducing the energy density of the diet has been shown to lower energy intakes. Four meta-analyses of weight change occurring on low-fat diets in intervention trials consistently demonstrate a highly significant weight loss of 3-4 kg in normal-weight and overweight subjects. The analyses also found a dose-response relationship, in other words the reduction in percentage energy as fat is positively associated with weight loss. Weight loss is also positively related to initial weight: a 10 % reduction in dietary fat is predicted to produce a 4-5 kg weight loss in an individual with a BMI of 30 kg/m^2 [48].

The greatest contributors to fat intake in the Irish diet are meats (23%), spreads (butter, margarine – 17%), cakes and biscuits (9%) and milk and yoghurt (9%) (Figure 2.2) [16].

Figure 2.2: Percentage contribution of foods to fat intake

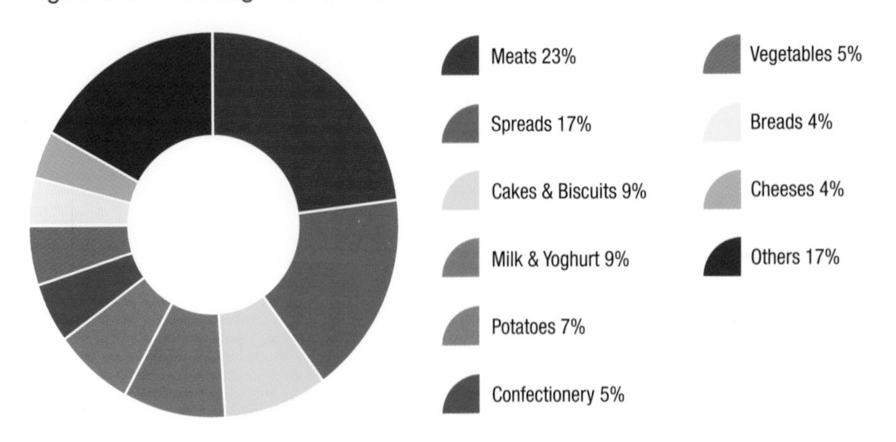

(Source: Irish Universities Nutrition Alliance, 2001)

Higher fat intakes can be compatible with health, but only if high physical activity is sustained throughout life. In sedentary societies, however, the inevitable seesaw between diet and physical activity leads to the conclusion that energy balance can only be achieved with less energy dense diets and with population average fat intakes of <30%[51].

Carbohydrate

With the increasing popularity of low-fat products, food intake statistics have shown a decrease in dietary fat intake, even though the prevalence of obesity is rising – the so called 'fat paradox'. A direct relationship between dietary fat and energy density has been questioned because many foods described as being 'low fat' or 'fat-free' are based on sugars, and thus they can have energy density values similar to those of their high-fat counterparts[52]. This has renewed interest in sugars as the primary nutritional factor behind the increase in obesity. **The World Health Organisation has published recommendations on daily sugar intake which acknowledge the link between sugar and weight gain**[42]. However, certain countries, such as the United States, do not refer directly to sugars in their guidelines because they require more evidence to support the link between sugary foods and weight gain; they include sugars with general carbohydrate recommendations.

Certain research evidence has shown that there is no direct link between high sugar consumption and increase in body mass index. Nevertheless, many refined carbohydrate foods produce a high glycaemic response, thereby promoting carbohydrate use in the body at the expense of fat. This means that the fat must be stored while the carbohydrate is being used[53]. This is in contrast to foods that produce a low glycaemic response and lower postprandial insulin‡ secretion. Research has suggested that a high intake of refined carbohydrates may increase the risk of insulin resistance leading to type 2 diabetes.

The percentage of energy from carbohydrate in the Irish population has increased since 1998. While there was a small increase in carbohydrate intake in men aged 35 to 54 the intakes increased by approximately 1% in women of all ages. Intakes of starch were lower in both males and females in 2002 but were higher in sugar intakes in all ages[47].

Bread contributes the most amount of carbohydrate energy from the Irish diet (25%) followed by potatoes (17%), cakes and biscuits (10%) and confectionery (10%) (Figure 2.3)[16].

Figure 2.3: Percentage contribution of foods to carbohydrate intake

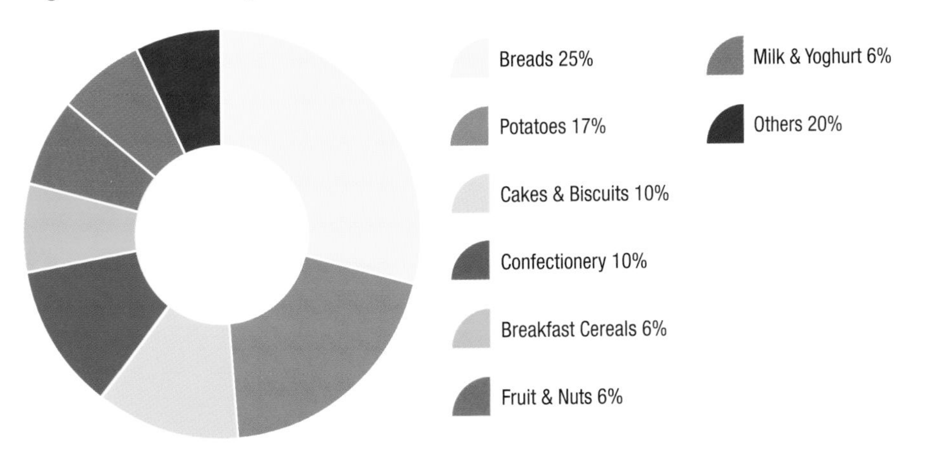

(Source: Irish Universities Nutrition Alliance, 2001)

‡ Insulin is a hormone that allows for the uptake of glucose (digested carbohydrate) into the cells for energy. Glucose is eventually converted to fat if it is not used as energy.

Fibre

High intakes of dietary fibre NSP (non-starch polysaccharide) are linked to the prevention and management of weight gain and obesity[55]. Under conditions of fixed energy intake, the majority of studies indicate that an increase in either soluble or insoluble fibre intake increases post-meal satiety and decreases subsequent hunger.

Intakes of fibre are generally lower in males and females over 55 years than in younger ages. Females had slightly higher intakes than males but there was little difference in intakes between 1998 and 2002[47].

Studies have also looked at other foods which do not seem to be associated with a raised BMI including plain rice and pasta, breakfast cereals, low fat spreads, soups and sauces, fruit, juices and nuts, fish, fish dishes and products[16].

Alcohol

Alcohol has the potential to promote weight gain because it is an energy dense nutrient. Energy ingested as alcohol is additional to energy from food. Alcohol consumption leads to a short-term increase in appetite which can increase energy intake. However on a long-term basis, moderate alcohol intake results in continual passive over-consumption[56].

There are two issues in relation to the evidence surrounding alcohol intake and increased weight gain. First, there is potential for confounding by lifestyle and socio-economic factors and there is a tendency to under-report alcohol intake[57]. Second, a poor understanding of the conversion of alcohol measures (pint/glass) to alcohol units could lead to an underestimation of the contribution of alcohol to energy intake. There is evidence to show that consumption of alcohol in Ireland continues to increase, ranking this country second highest in Europe per head of population[58].

Compliance with recommendations

Compliance with the Irish Food Pyramid recommendations has changed in the last few years. The Cereals, Bread and Potatoes shelf was the only shelf which showed a decrease in compliance with food pyramid recommendations over the past four years[47]. All shelves showed modest increases in compliance (Figure 2.4). The Fruit and Vegetable shelf had the highest increase in compliance, particularly among men[47].

Figure 2.4: Percentage compliance with shelves of the pyramid by gender

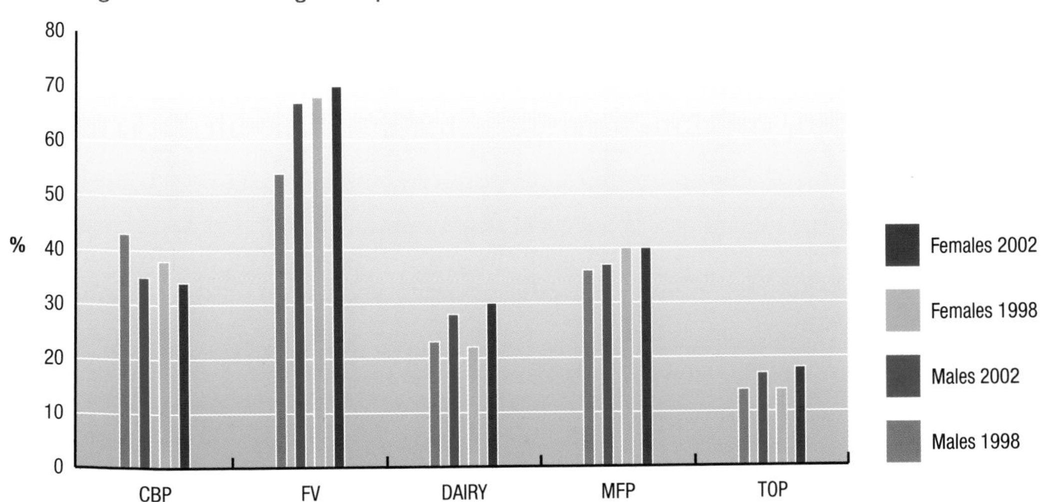

CBP = cereals, bread, potatoes
FV = fruit and vegetables
DAIRY = milk, cheese, yoghurt
MFP = meat, fish, poultry and other protein alternatives
TOP = foods that are high in fat and/or salt and/or sugar

Food prepared outside the home

Increasing demands on time due for example to work commitments and commuting distances has led to an increasing demand for pre-prepared food that is readily available to the home or food prepared outside the home. In Ireland this is noticeable in the proliferation of deli or fast-food counters in petrol station forecourts and convenience supermarkets. While fruit, vegetables and other healthier options are also available the desire for ready-made foods/foods prepared outside the home means that they are often overlooked in favour of more energy dense foods. In the United States, the energy, total fat, saturated fat, cholesterol and sodium content of foods prepared outside the home is significantly higher than that of home-prepared food[59]. Americans who tend to eat in restaurants have a higher BMI than those who tend to eat at home[60]. The British now eat more fast-food than any other country in Western Europe and the fast-food sector has been projected to expand by 30% over the next ten years [61].

The majority of the population do not eat out in expensive restaurants on a regular basis but 19% consume food from work canteens, 12% from inexpensive restaurants, 15% from cafes, 10% from fast-food outlets, and 6% use home delivery services at least once a week (SLÁN, 2002). In general men tend to consume more food prepared outside the home. The highest consumers of food prepared outside the home are males and females aged between 18 and 34 (Figure 2.5).

Figure 2.5: Percentage eating out once a week/not most days by age group

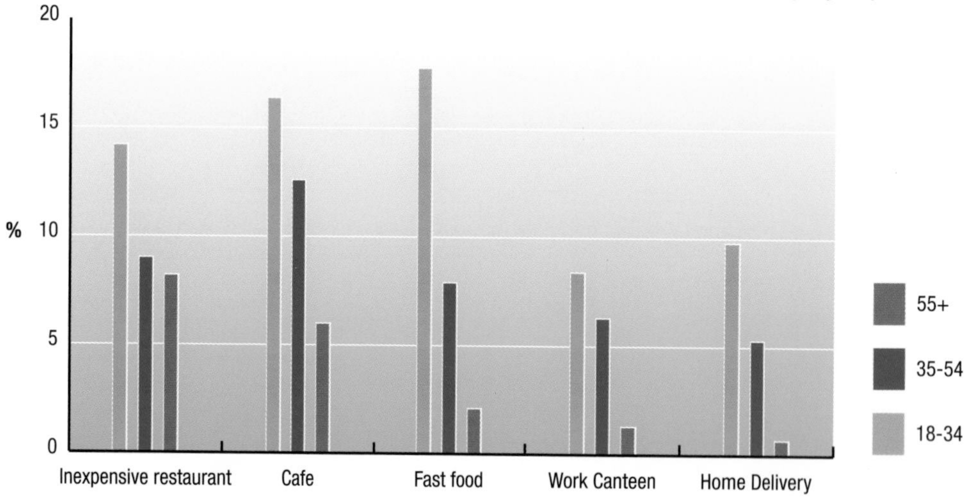

(Source: SLÁN, 2002)

Inexpensive restaurants, cafes and fast-food outlets are frequented on a weekly basis (Figure 2.5). Work canteens are the main source of food consumed outside the home on a daily basis. As many as 22.2% of 18 to 34 year-olds and 13% of 35 to 54 year-olds use work canteens on a daily basis (Figure 2.6).

Figure 2.6: Percentage eating out every day/most days by age group

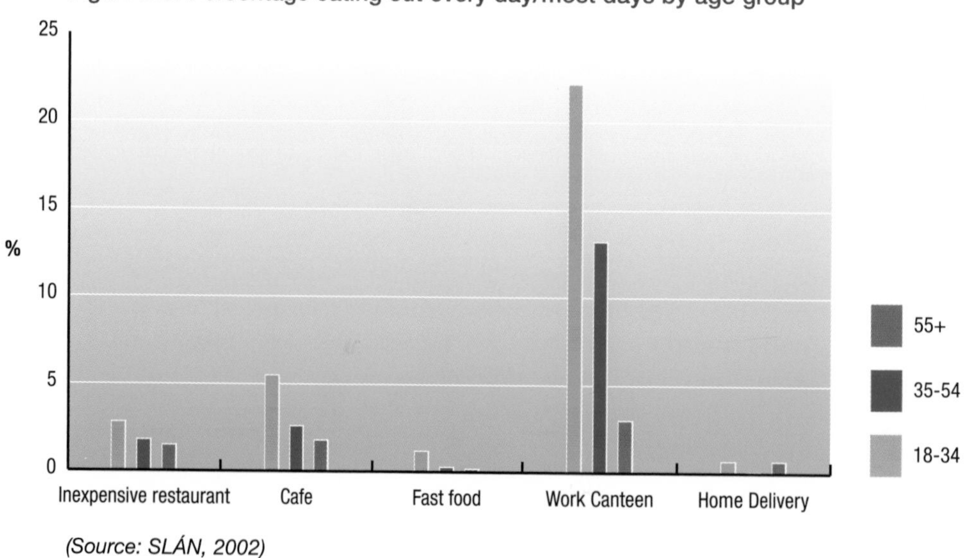

(Source: SLÁN, 2002)

The North/South Ireland Food Consumption Survey found a similar age trend in the percentage of energy derived from food and drink 'eaten out', with males obtaining more energy from these food sources than females (Figure 2.7)[16].

Figure 2.7: Percentage of total energy from foods/drinks 'eaten out'

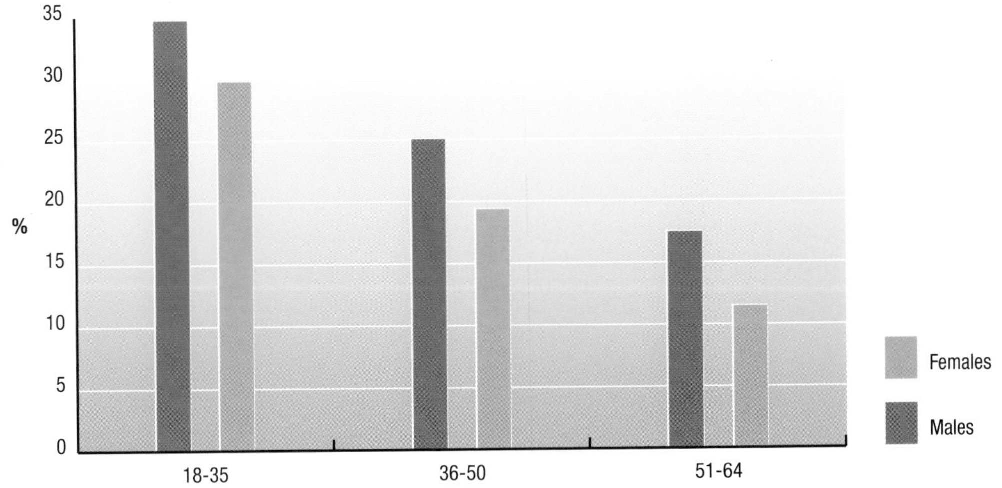

(Source: Irish Universities Nutrition Alliance, 2001)

Children's dietary habits

Children are consuming large amounts of energy dense foods which may be provided in or outside the home. **The recent HBSC 2002 survey showed that 51% of Irish children consumed sweets, 37% drank fizzy drinks, 27% consumed crisps, 12% ate chips and 7% ate hamburgers at least once daily** (Figure 2.8)[62]. Among children aged 10 to 17, 42.9% of boys and 33% of girls consumed a fizzy drink at least once a day. Sweets were consumed daily or more by 48.9% of boys and 52.7% of girls. These foods were consumed more frequently by the older children (15-17). Foods that are high in fat and salt – crisps, hamburgers and chips – were consumed more by the younger aged girls (10-11) and boys aged 10-11 and 12-14 years [62].

Figure 2.8: Energy dense food consumption patterns in Irish children

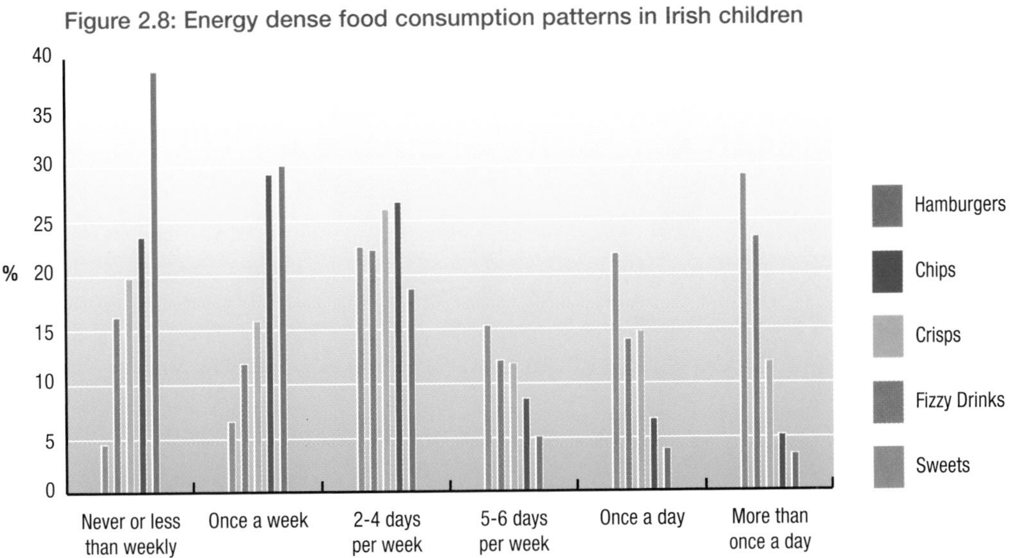

(Source: HBSC, 2003)

The World Health Organisation has serious concerns over the high and increasing consumption of sugar-sweetened drinks by children in many countries[42]. Sugar-sweetened carbonated drinks seem to be a contributory factor to the obesity epidemic[63]. Children who drink one regular carbonated drink a day have an average 10% more total energy than non-consumers[64]. It has been estimated that each additional can or glass of sugar-sweetened drink that children consume every day increases the risk of becoming obese by 60%[65]. Most of the research relates to carbonated drinks but many fruit drinks and cordials are equally energy-dense and may promote weight gain if consumed in large quantities.

The Department of Health and Children has provided food and nutrition guidelines for primary schools and preschools. There is a statutory obligation on pre-school providers (i) to ensure that suitable, sufficient, nutritious and varied food is available for pre-school children attending a pre-school service on a full-time basis and (ii) to provide adequate and suitable facilities for indoor and outdoor play taking account of numbers of children, their age and the amount of time spent in the service. Pre-school services are inspected by the pre-school inspection service of the HSE against both requirements. The revised Pre-School Regulations due to be published later this year will place a greater emphasis on the importance of play in child development and on children's physical well-being.

Portion sizes

Large portion sizes are a possible causative factor for unhealthy weight gain[42]. Between 1977 and 1998 the energy intake and portion size of salty snacks increased by 93 kcal (28.4 to 45.4 g), soft drinks by 49 kcal (387.4 to 588.4 ml), hamburgers by 97 kcal (161.6 to 198.4 g), French fries by 68 kcal (87.9 to 102.1 g)[66]. According to WHO there is some evidence that people poorly estimate portion sizes and that subsequent energy compensation for a large meal is incomplete and therefore is likely to lead to over-consumption (WHO, 2003)[42].

Portion sizes have been shown to have an influence on weight gain. The North-South Ireland Food Consumption Survey showed that consuming large fries as opposed to regular fries on a regular basis could give 5.7:1 odds of becoming obese. The likelihood of being obese compared to normal weight was increased 3.9 times by consumption of 'high calorie' beverages compared to 'low calorie' beverages[67].

Dietary restraint

Dietary restraint and disinhibition are two of three psychological constructs of eating behaviour. Dietary restraint is defined as the tendency to restrict the amount or types of foods consumed for the purpose of maintaining or losing weight. Dietary disinhibition can be defined as the tendency to over-eat certain foods with characteristics that one finds appealing (for example palatability) or in response to disinhibiting stimuli (for example at a buffet, during emotional distress or alcohol consumption).

Restraint relates to body size through its interaction with disinhibition. Dietary restraint scores increase and disinhibition and hunger scores decrease with weight loss whereas maintenance of weight loss is associated with higher restraint and lower disinhibition and hunger scores. Greater disinhibition is associated with greater weight gain, even after controlling for confounding factors[68]. Individuals with high disinhibition and any level of restraint are heavier and larger than those with low levels of disinhibition. High disinhibition coupled with low levels of restraint is associated with the greatest weight and size[69].

More women (19.8%) follow weight-reducing diets than men (5%)(Figure 2.9). The number of women following weight-reducing diets has increased since 1998: it has decreased for men[28].

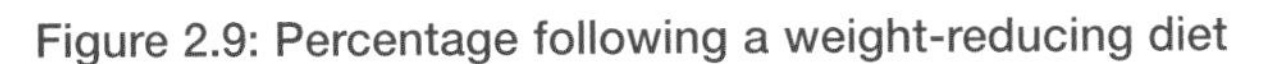

Figure 2.9: Percentage following a weight-reducing diet

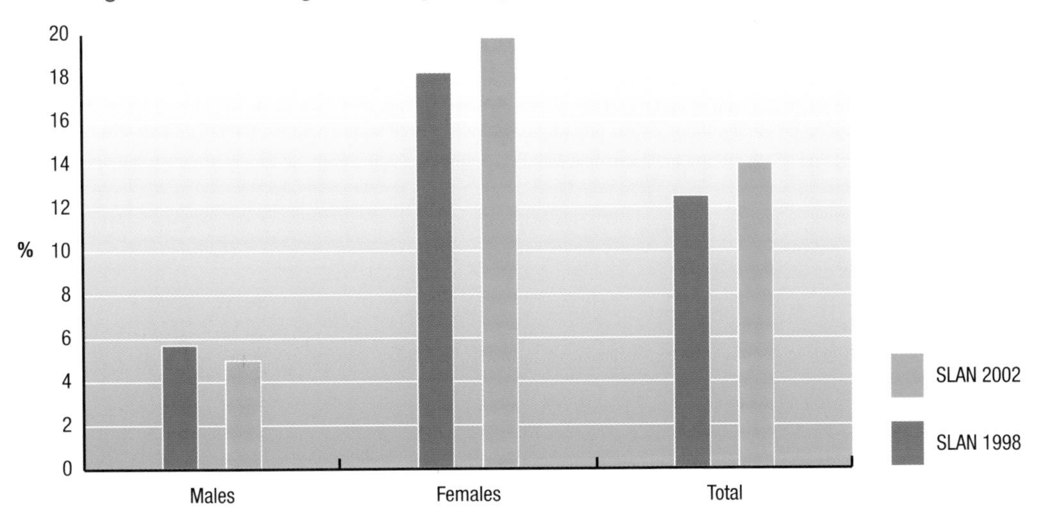

(Source: SLÁN, 2003)

The number of children following weight-reducing diets has increased since 1998. The percentage of girls following these diets is higher than that of 12 to 14 year-old and 15 to 17 year-old boys. However, similar percentages of boys and girls aged 10 to 11 report following weight-reduction diets (Figure 2.10 and Figure 2.11)[28].

Figure 2.10: Percentage of boys who report being on a weight-reducing diet

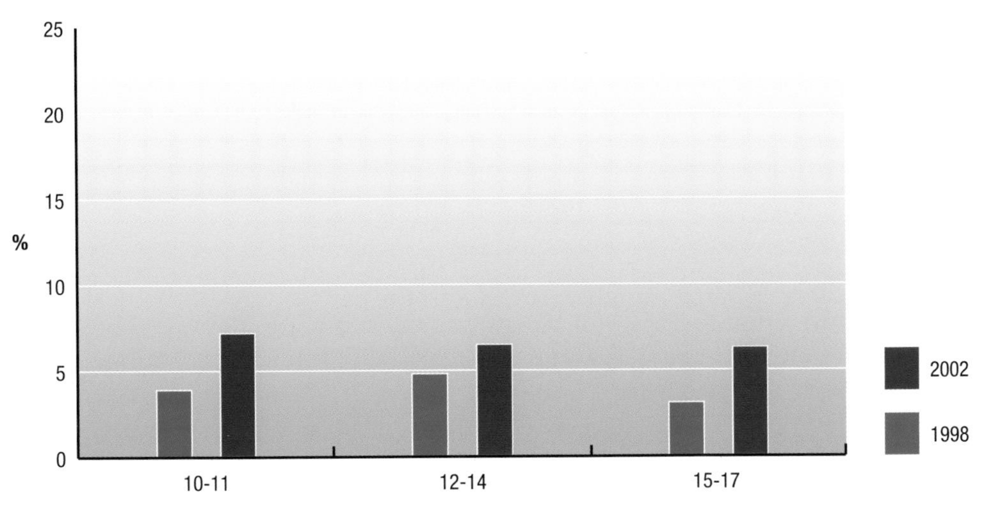

(Source: HBSC, 2003)

Figure 2.11: Percentage of girls who report being on a weight-reducing diet

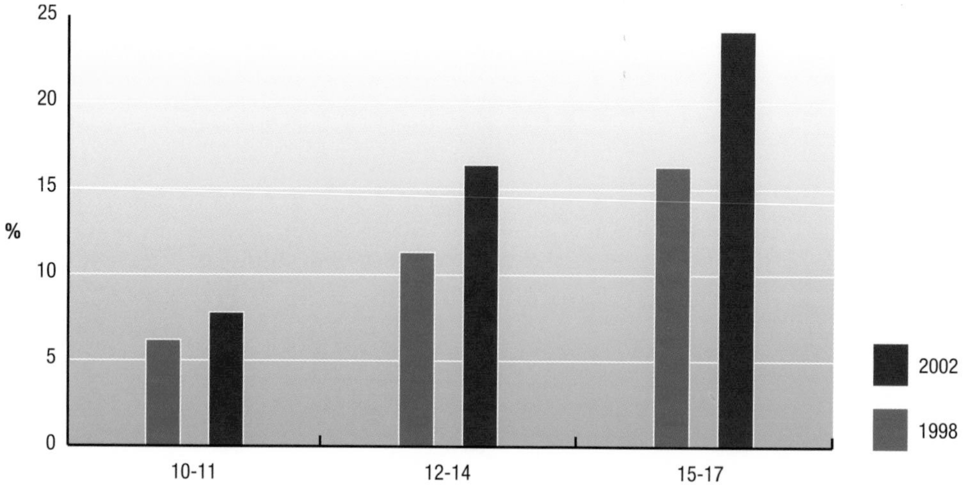

(Source: HBSC, 2003)

In another Irish survey, fifth class children were asked if they had ever tried to lose weight, and whether they were trying to lose weight at the time of the survey[70]. The response was 17% of boys and 20% of girls had tried to lose weight and 10% of boys and 15% of girls were trying to lose weight at the time of the survey. The most frequently employed method among boys and girls were 'exercise' and 'cutting out sweets', while 'fasting' and 'eating less food' were also mentioned. A study of Dublin school children also found that significantly more girls than boys were affected by fear of fatness and were trying to loose weight[39].

The relationship between unhealthy weight-loss practices and smoking is a particular cause for concern. Lower levels of overweight and obesity are prevalent among smokers[71]. A study of Dublin schoolgirls found that almost 20% of girls 'starting' or 'continuing to smoke' used it as a weight-loss strategy[72].

Breastfeeding

Evidence is accumulating that early infancy may be a critical period for the development of obesity. Several studies have identified rapid weight gain during the first six months of life as a determinant of overweight during childhood[73, 74] and young adulthood[75]. These associations are important considering that rapid growth during early infancy was identified in as many as 29% of babies in one of the cohort studies[75]. However, apart from encouragement of breastfeeding, safe and effective interventions in early infancy for the prevention of obesity are not well established. **Research has shown that breastfeeding exclusively for a) at least two months seems to be protective against the development of overweight in childhood[76] and b) for six months seems to be protective against the development of overweight during adolescence[77].** Possible mechanisms for a protective effect of breastfeeding include the slower growth rates of breastfed babies compared with formula-fed babies after the first two months of life. This probably relates to the relative control breastfed babies compared with formula-fed babies can exert over their energy intake[77].

Breastfeeding confers many other long-term and short-term health benefits to both mother and baby. Therefore, for prevention of obesity, encouragement of exclusive breastfeeding for the first six months of life if possible, represents the only known safe intervention that can be implemented in early infancy [77,76,42,57].

Possible genetic predisposition

Historically, the survival of the human species depends on its ability to adapt to its changing environment and this is reflected through a very gradual change in the genotype of many generations[78]. The tendency to store energy in the form of fat is believed to result from thousands of years of evolution in an environment characterised by poor food supplies. This is know as the 'thrifty genotype' whereby those who could store energy in times of plenty were more likely to survive periods of famine and to pass this tendency to their offspring[79]. However in a modern environment this tendency predisposes the individual to an increased risk of obesity.

Obesity and overweight result from an imbalance between caloric intake and relative physical activity that is modulated by a susceptible genotype. Individuals with a family history of obesity may be predisposed to gain weight. Evidence from twin, adoption and family studies strongly suggests that biological relatives exhibit similarities in maintenance of body weight.

Obese individuals have genetic similarities that may shed light on the biological differences that predispose to weight gain. For instance exceptional mutations of the leptin gene and its receptor have been described in obese individuals. These genes encode proteins that are strongly connected to the regulation of food intake. This knowledge may be useful in preventing or treating obesity in predisposed people.

While there are rare obesity syndromes caused by mutations in single genes, by far the greatest proportion of obesity in humans is not due to mutations in single genes. Genetic variations in individuals can produce different responses when the individual interacts with his or her environment.

In the longer term, understanding the genetic variations that influence energy metabolism may help us to understand the underlying biological factors that affect weight gain and energy expenditure and may lead to interventions that capitalise on these insights. Fat stores are regulated over long periods of time by complex systems that involve input and feedback from fatty tissues, the brain and endocrine glands like the pancreas and the thyroid. Overweight and obesity can result from only a very small positive energy input imbalance over a long period of time.

The rapid changes which are taking place however, for example in the numbers of obese children within a relatively stable population, indicate that genetic factors are not the primary reason for change[32].

WHO summary

A review carried out by Swinburn and colleagues on behalf of the Joint WHO/FAO Expert Consultation on diet, nutrition and the prevention of chronic diseases provides an overview of the principle dietary factors related to the development of weight gain and obesity[42,57] (Table 2.2). The review does not examine in detail other lifestyle factors, apart from dietary ones, which may influence overweight and obesity.

Table 2.2: Summary of strength of evidence on factors that might promote or protect against weight gain and obesity

Evidence[1]	Decreased risk	No relationship	Increased risk
Convincing	Regular physical activity		Sedentary lifestyles
	High dietary intake of NSP[2] (fibre)		High intake of energy-dense, micronutrient poor foods
Probable	Home and school environments that support healthy food choices for children		Heavy marketing of energy-dense foods and fast-food outlets
	Breastfeeding		High intake of sugar-sweetened soft drinks and juices Adverse socio-economic conditions
Possible	Low glycaemic index foods	Protein content of diet	Large portion sizes
			High proportions of food prepared outside the home Rigid restraint/periodic disinhibition eating patterns (diets)
Insufficient	Increased eating frequency		Alcohol

1. Definitions of the levels of evidence can be found in Appendix C

2. NSP – Non-starch polysaccharide

PHYSICAL ACTIVITY

Physical activity is an important determinant of body weight. There is a general move away from physically demanding work. This, together with the increasing use of automated transport, technology in the home, and more passive leisure time all contribute to lower levels of physical activity.

Physical activity is defined as 'bodily movement produced by the contraction of skeletal muscle that increases energy expenditure above the basal level'. Physical activity can be categorised in various ways, including type, intensity, and purpose[80]. Exercise is generally defined as 'physical activity that is planned, structured, repetitive, and purposive in the sense that improvement or maintenance of one or more components of physical fitness is the objective'[81]. Physical activity and exercise are two terms that are often used interchangeably, but it is important to make a distinction between them. While they are similar in nature, it is now agreed that exercise falls within the more broad definition of physical activity.

Energy expenditure and physical activity

Energy is utilised to maintain the functional integrity of organs and tissues in the body and to sustain physiological processes, including respiration, blood distribution, digestion and absorption, muscle contraction, growth, temperature regulation and physical work. Basal energy expenditure refers to the minimum amount of energy required to sustain life. This is a relatively constant rate of expenditure but can be influenced by body size, physical fitness and energy intake. Daily physical activity is more variable than basal energy expenditure and is influenced by the physical environment, the social environment, and by cultural and lifestyle factors. Because physical activity accounts for the greatest variability in energy expenditure, dietary intake should be reflective of activity level. **The increase in sedentary lifestyles, the decrease in work-related physical activity, and reduced leisure-time activity suggest that physical inactivity has made a significant impact on the increase in overweight and obesity being seen today**[82].

The biological need for physical activity

From an evolutionary perspective, the human genome has evolved to support physical activity and has changed relatively little since the emergence of early Homo sapiens. Until the relatively recent advent of industrialised societies our ancestors lived and evolved in a physically demanding environment. The high level of daily physical activity was largely responsible for the expression of genes regulating metabolism, energy expenditure and substrate utilisation [83]. While this regulation of metabolism has changed little, daily physical activity in modern society has decreased. The failure to stimulate gene expression by physical activity has contributed to altered metabolic regulation and an increase in hypokinetic diseases including obesity, type 2 diabetes, cardiovascular disease, cancer and osteoporosis.

The trends in physical activity

Data from a number of countries suggest that a large proportion of people are not meeting the recommended level of physical activity for general health benefits, and even fewer achieve the target to prevent weight gain. The longitudinal monitoring of physical activity has not been comprehensive but these data also suggest that physical activity levels have been in decline across all age groups[84].

European Union data

In 2003 the Eurobarometer survey looked at physical activity patterns and trends within the European Union. One of the questions asked was: 'In the last seven days, how many days did you do physical activity?' Those reporting no vigorous physical activity ranged from 43% in the Netherlands to 72 % in Spain. Other countries that reported having low rates of vigorous physical activity were Italy 64%, Ireland 62% and Belgium 61%[85]. The most active countries in the EU were Sweden, Austria and Finland where over 40% were physically active five hours a week or more. Consistent with United States findings, it was also found that within the EU those with more education are more physically active[85]. Overall within Europe between 5% and 8 % of deaths are attributable to physical inactivity[86].

In the UK 30% of the boys and 51% of the girls in the 7-10 age group were not achieving the recommended one hour per day of moderate exercise, and these numbers increased in the 15-18 age group[87]. A study commissioned by Sport England showed that the percentage of young people engaging in physical activity for more than two hours per week decreased from 46% in 1994 to 33% in 1999[88]. There was a fall in the number of children walking and cycling to school, while the proportion of students being driven to school had increased[89].

United States data

In the United States approximately 15% of US adults engage in vigorous physical activity (three times a week for twenty minutes) and between 25%[80] to 40%[90] of US adults reported no physical activity at all. Another recent US study showed that the vast majority of adolescents were not achieving thirty minutes of physical activity per day, and this trend was continued into adulthood[90]. Only 19% of high school students in the US reported being physically active for twenty minutes or more daily and 14% reported having engaged in no physical activity at all[80].

Irish Data

The National Health and Lifestyle Surveys[28] conducted in 1998 and 2002 reflect a representative cross-section of the Irish population. Information on physical activity levels in both adults and children were collected in 1998 and 2002, to allow for a comprehensive investigation of changes in physical activity of the Irish population.

Adults

In 2002, 51% (52% in 1998) of the Irish adult population reported engaging in some form of physical activity, 22% performing mild exercise four or more times per week, 32% doing moderate exercise three or more times per week, and 11% engaging in strenuous exercise three or more times per week[28]. There were strong trends according to educational status, age and physical activity, with those having more education reporting more physical activity. Those who spend more time sitting, who are not physically active in their job and those who perform mild exercise only are more likely to be obese. In contrast, those who do regular light housework, and engage in regular moderate or strenuous activity are less likely to be obese[28].

Although there was no statistically significant changes in adults participating in physical activity between 1998 and 2002 (Figure 2.12) there were statistically significant (at the 0.001 level) differences with age, with participation in physical activity decreasing with age.

Figure 2.12: Percentages of adults engaged in regular exercise by age group

100
80
60
40
20
0
%
Males
Females
55+ years 2002
35-54 years 2002
18-34 years 2002
55+ years 1998
35-54 years 1998
18-34 years 1998

(Source: SLÁN, 2003)

Those reporting no exercise by age group (Figure 2.13) showed an increase in the 35-54 year-old males from 20% to 28% and in the 55+ year-old males from 34% to 46%. In the females all the age groups reported an increase with the 18 to 34 year-olds going from 12% to 16%, the 35-54 year-old females from 16% to 19%, and the 55+ year-old females from 38% to 46%. Again those reporting no activity increased with age[28].

Figure 2.13: Percentages of adults engaged in no exercise by age group

100
80
60
40
20
0
%
Males
Females
55+ years 2002
35-54 years 2002
18-34 years 2002
55+ years 1998
35-54 years 1998
18-34 years 1998

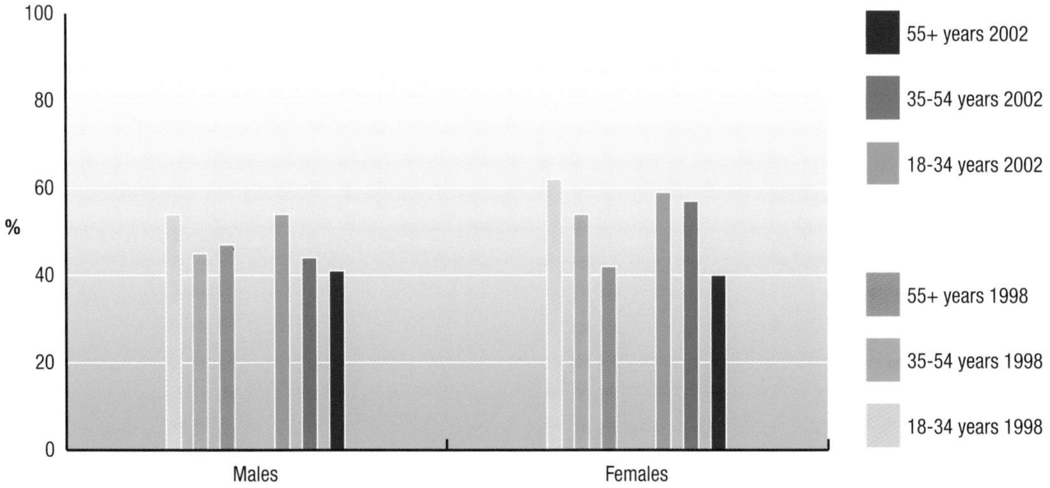

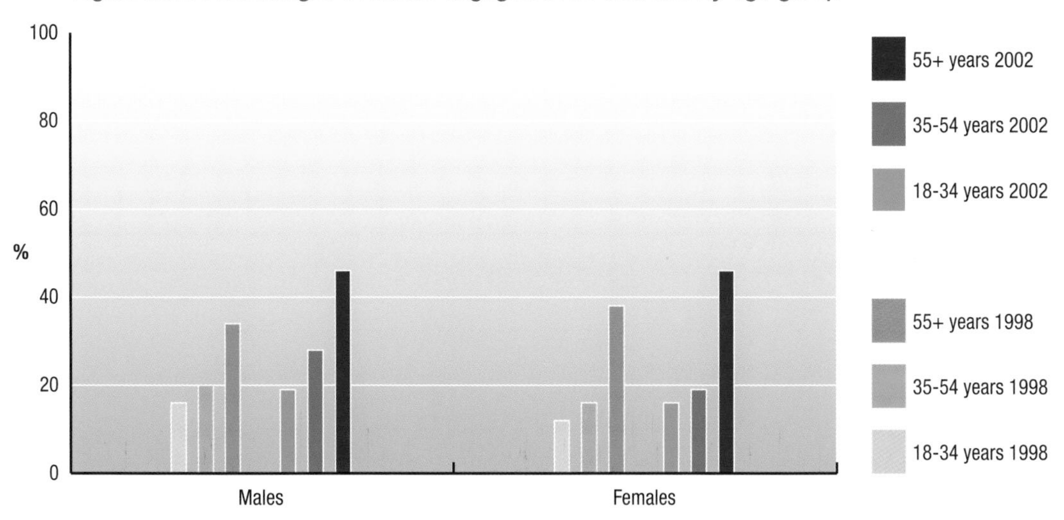

(Source: SLÁN, 2003)

Children and adolescents

According to the Health Behaviour in School-Aged Children survey data [28] from 1998 and 2002 (Figure 2.14 and Figure 2.15), the only children to change their physical activity levels significantly were 12 to 14 year-old girls within the vigorous activity level group. This age group decreased from 49% in 1998 to 44% in 2002. **Physical activity levels decrease with age and there is normally a significant change after adolescence.** This is a significant finding because the drop is occurring at a younger age. The information is important for policy makers and health promotion professionals because the middle school years are an important time in which to intervene[91].

Figure 2.14: Percentages of boys engaged in vigorous exercise outside school hours

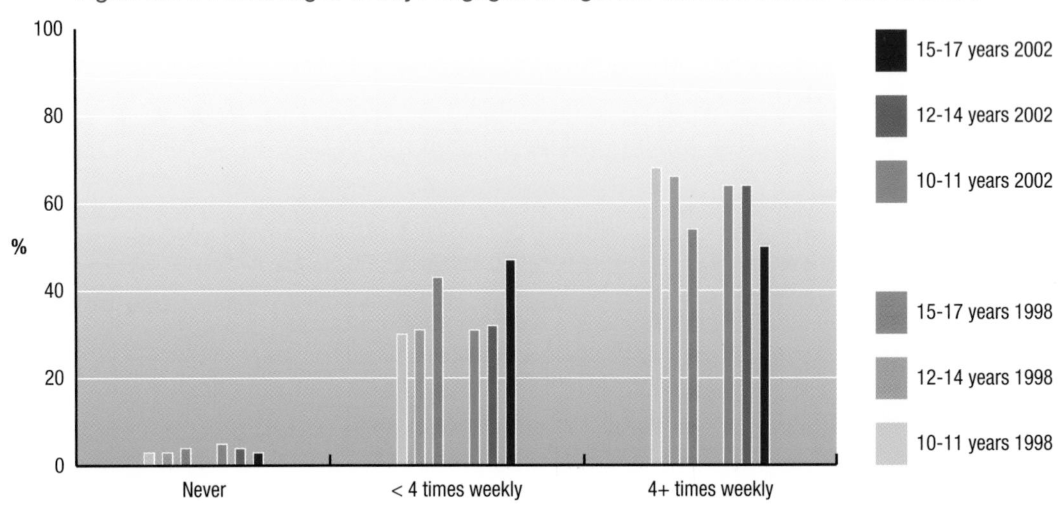

(Source: HBSC, 2003)

Figure 2.15: Percentages of girls engaged in vigorous exercise outside school hours

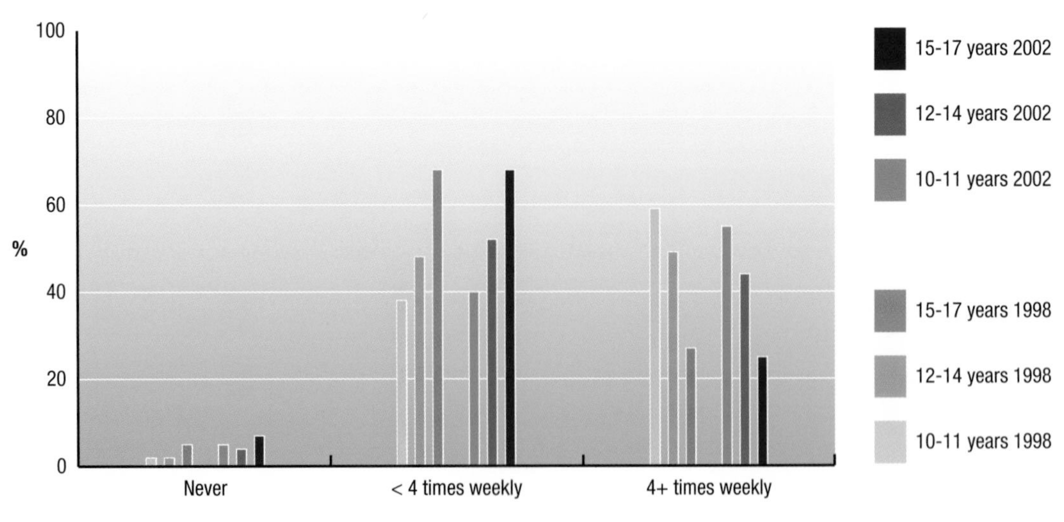

(Source: HBSC, 2003)

There were significant increases in the reported levels of no physical activity and physical activity less than weekly. The inactivity rates were higher in the girls with a sharp increase after the age of fifteen[28]. There were no consistent significant relationships between physical activity and social class found in the children's age groups.

Take Part Study

The aim of the Take PART (Physical Activity Research for Teenagers) Study[92] was to i) assess fitness levels, ii) develop an understanding of the participation levels in physical activity, and iii) increase research knowledge in exercise behaviour modification in young people. The participants were 15 to 17 year-olds within the East Coast Area Health Board (ECAHB) region. Various psycho-social and physical measurements were collected.

- A total of 65% of participants were not involved in moderate or vigorous physical activity for > 4 days for at least 60 minutes per day. The amount of subjects not regularly active for > 5 days was 80%.
- The 65% not regularly active had significantly lower aerobic fitness levels and lower minutes of participation in leisure-time physical activity than their regularly active counterparts.
- Females were significantly less likely to be physically active and had a lower level of aerobic fitness compared to a similar age-group in Northern Ireland[93].
- Individuals with high BMI had correspondingly low levels of leisure-time physical activity and aerobic fitness (Figure 2.16).
- Unhealthy lifestyle choices and extreme weight management decisions were more likely to be made by obese or overweight individuals. They were however not uncommon amongst normal weight adolescents.

Figure 2.16: Aerobic fitness according to BMI and gender

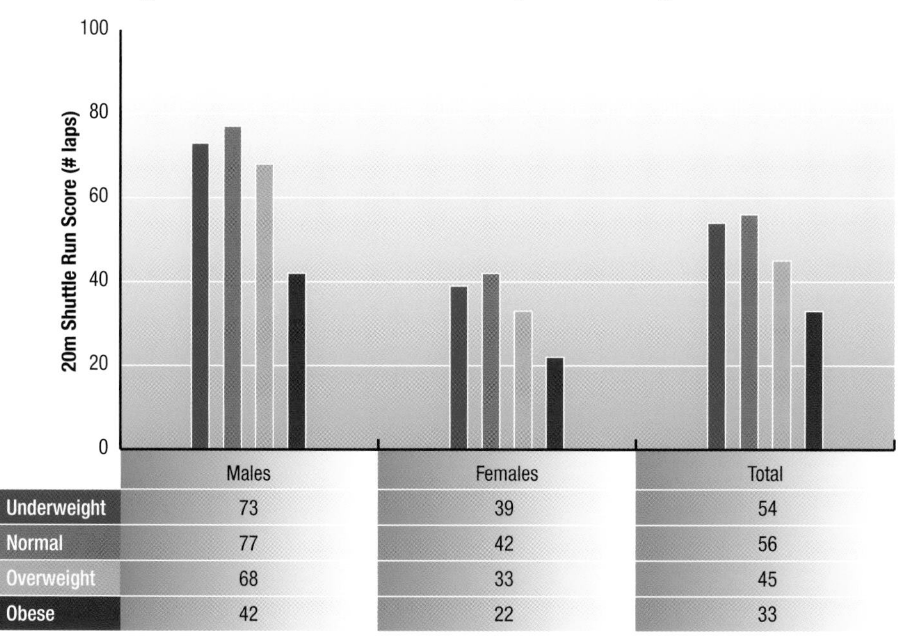

	Males	Females	Total
Underweight	73	39	54
Normal	77	42	56
Overweight	68	33	45
Obese	42	22	33

The majority of participants (61%) travelled to school by motorised transport, with no difference between males and females. Of these, 22% of car users and 3% of bus users travelled less than or equal to one mile to school. **Obese adolescents were more than twice as likely to have a high incidence of sedentary leisure habits compared to normal or overweight adolescents.** There was a high rate of reported television viewing with 70% of males and 60% of females viewing two or more hours daily of television[92].

Mid-Western Region Heart Rate Monitoring Study

A heart rate monitoring study in a second-level school in the mid-western region of Ireland found that none of the study participants were active for >30 minutes of moderate intensity (>140 bpm) cumulative physical activity on all four days[94]. No adolescents in the study had three or more sustained twenty-minute periods of vigorous physical activity. The females in this study were consistently less active than the males in all the physical activity levels on any day of measurement[94].

Television viewing

Several large studies have documented associations between numbers of hours of television viewed and both the prevalence and incidence of obesity. The IUNA study found that BMI and waist circumference increased as time spent viewing television increased[95]. People of normal weight spend less time watching television and more time carrying out vigorous physical activity[95].

Studies have shown that television viewing, playing video games for long periods of time, or not participating in sports outside of school, promotes obesity in children[96]. One study has shown that television alone is not independently related to an increase in BMI in children[97]. The combination of lifestyle factors that accompany lengthy television use appears to place children at risk of obesity and poor nutritional status[98].

Research carried out by the Broadcasting Commission of Ireland[99] found that children aged 4 to 14 years watched an average of 2.72 hours of television per day. The percentage of Irish adolescents watching television on weekdays and weekends tends to be lower than that of the International HBSC average[100]. While all children tend to watch more television at weekends, more boys than girls reported longer sessions of television viewing throughout the week (Figure 2.17 and Figure 2.18)[100]. According to a recent survey of children in first class in Cork city, 22% of 7 and 8 year-olds watch three or more hours of television each weekday and 50% watch three or more hours at weekends[101]. This study also reported that one-third of children in first class had a television set in their bedroom.

Fig 2.17: Percentage of young people who watch television ≥ 4 hours per day on weekdays

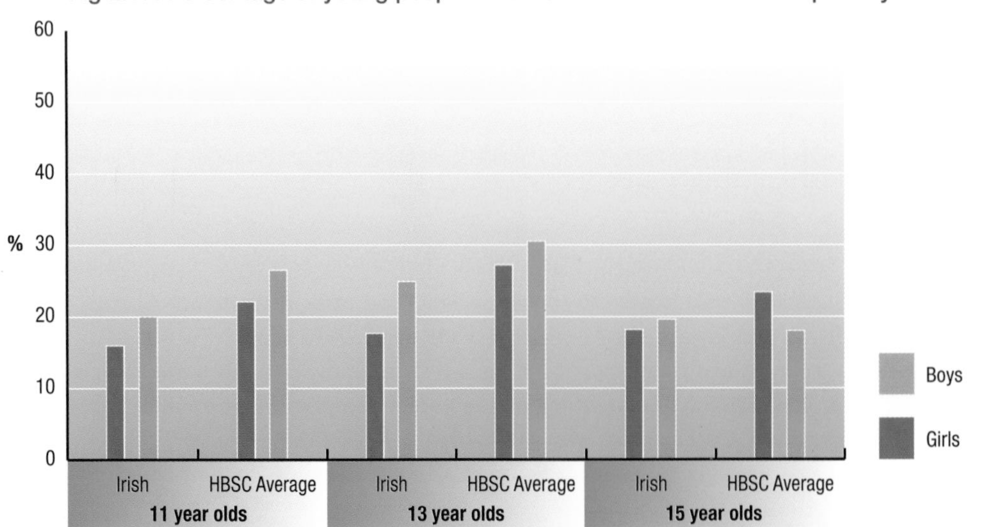

Fig 2.18: Percentage of young people who watch television ≥ 4 hours per day at weekends

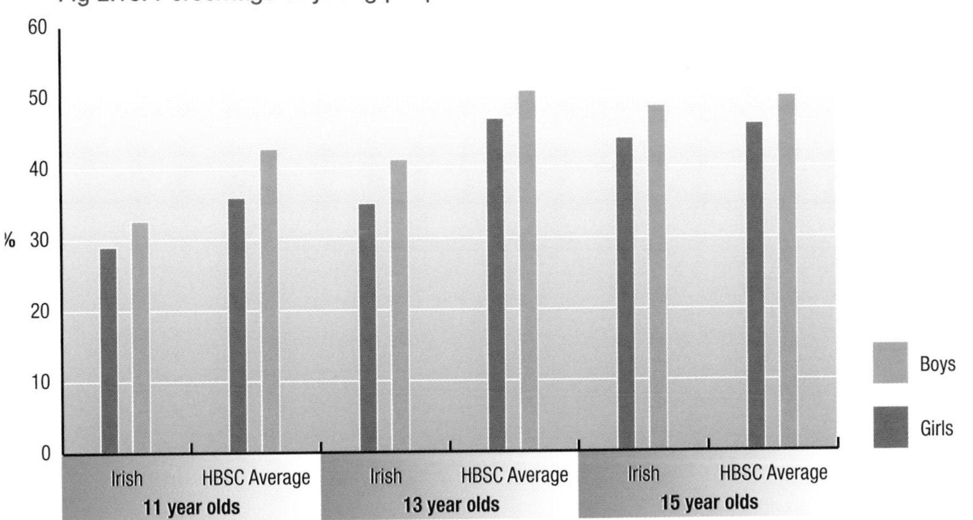

How much physical activity is enough?

There has been a lot of confusion regarding recommendations for physical activity. In the last decade recommendations have been largely based on a desire to reduce cardiovascular disease mortality and improve general health. In our society, which has increasing demands on time, the recommendations have leaned towards the least amount of physical activity required to show a protective effect.

In the 1990s the American College of Sports Medicine (ACSM) recommended that we should 'accumulate at least 30 minutes or more of moderate-intensity physical activity on most, preferably all days of the week'. While the ACSM was careful to stress the requirement of 'at least 30-minutes', many countries around the world have adopted the target of 30-minutes physical activity. While there is substantial evidence to support the health-related benefits of achieving and maintaining this recommendation, it has emerged that this level of physical activity may not be adequate to prevent excess weight gain.

The International Association for the Study of Obesity (IASO) consensus statement from its First Stock Conference indicated that **45-60 minutes of moderate intensity activity is required to prevent the transition to overweight or obesity**[102].This recommendation was supported by a report from the United States Institute of Medicine (IoM) who recommended 60-minutes of physical activity per day to prevent excess weight gain and **between 60-90 minutes per day for weight loss and the maintenance of weight loss.** This recommendation came from a comprehensive analysis of studies that measured total daily energy expenditure by doubly labelled water and other epidemiological studies.

There is now a wider acceptance of the need to review physical activity recommendations for the prevention of weight gain and the treatment of overweight/obesity. The Chief Medical Officer in the UK has recently differentiated between physical activity recommendations for general health and those for the prevention of weight gain. These recommendations are in line with the IASO and the IoM.

In regard to children and young people it has been even more difficult to present adequate physical activity recommendations. It is generally accepted that **children should be involved in at least 60 minutes of moderate physical activity each day.** It is difficult to obtain objective longitudinal data on this population and with the recent rapid increase in childhood obesity, these recommendations may also be revised.

The intensity and duration of physical activity

One of the other difficulties in interpreting physical activity recommendations has been the intensity of effort required. While there is some evidence to demonstrate a greater benefit from vigorous intensity exercise, other data suggest that overall daily energy expenditure is most important, irrespective of intensity. The recommendations outlined above would equate to approximately **2.4-3.4 MJ (500-700 kcal) expenditure per day**. Therefore, if the intensity of physical activity was vigorous, it would be possible to achieve this goal in a shorter period of time. It would also be possible to expend 2.4-3.4 MJ by active daily living but the overall duration required may exceed 60 minutes.

3 The COST to SOCIETY

KEY POINTS

- Obesity can lead to stigma, prejudice, low self-esteem, isolation and humiliation.
- The cost for treating obesity in Ireland is estimated at €0.4 billion.
- The number of premature deaths annually attributable to obesity currently approximates to 2,000.
- As much as 58% of type 2 diabetes, 21% of heart disease and between 8% and 42% of certain cancers are attributable to excess body fat.

3 The COST to SOCIETY

When Ireland was a much poorer country and there was widespread undernourishment and even starvation, the ideal for any person was to be well fed and looking well fed was therefore symbolic of higher social status – something desirable and to be envied. The health consequences of being overfed outweighed those of undernutrition. This created the attitude, for instance among mothers and others, that a healthy baby was a baby that was and looked overweight – the fat bonny baby.

These attitudes to health are now completely outdated, yet we are developing a generation of overweight children and adults. Being overweight now has many individual health consequences but of equal or more importance are the social consequences of a society where overweight and obesity has become the norm. This may be the first generation where children will have lower life expectancy than their parents, leaving a huge social gap in family relationships and caring for older family members.

Much of everyday social contact depends on sharing space with others, space that has been developed to accommodate average sizes. This explains why overweight people no longer fit into theatre and cinema seats, train or aeroplane seats – with associated costs of change. As children and then as adults overweight people have suffered negative attitudes and stigma at an individual level but in increasing numbers and therefore with increasing costs to society. This has led to more obvious and ingrained discrimination in the workplace, at school and in leisure facilities.

The increase in overweight and obesity has the potential to disrupt many of our social patterns and interactions: increased illness will negate the achievements of medical advances; decreased productivity will affect economic balance and reduce competitiveness and the ability to pay society's costs for pensions and benefits; increased demand for foodstuffs will affect the markets and the demand-supply economy; social behaviours and attitudes will reflect the increased prevalence of overweight and there will be an increase in prejudice against obese individuals.

SOCIAL IMPACT OF OBESITY

Obese people are at an increased risk of developing many medical problems. Overweight and obesity carry serious implications for psychosocial health, mainly due to prejudice against fatness, particularly female fatness, which is widespread[103]. Being obese is considered as indicative of a loss of self-control, a 'risk' for ill-health and a problem to be corrected. This gives rise to considerable social stigma, low self-esteem, isolation and humiliation.

Among adults in industrialised countries, research demonstrates the social and economic effects of obesity. A study by Gortmaker et al (1993) found that obese adults are more likely to live in poverty, are less educated, less likely to earn as much and less likely to date or marry than their non-overweight counterparts[104]. The disadvantages attributed to being obese were found to be of a lesser magnitude in men.

Prejudice and discrimination

Prejudice and discrimination towards obese individuals persist despite worldwide increases in the prevalence of obesity and the recognition that genetics can be a factor for some individuals. **Ridicule and disparagement of obese individuals seems to remain a socially acceptable form of prejudice**[105]. There is evidence of clear and consistent weight prejudice in areas of life such as employment, healthcare and education[106]. Bias has been documented among employers and co-workers, teachers, nurses, physicians, mental health professionals, landlords, peers, multiple media sources, parents, and children as young as age three[107]. Given that existing weight-loss approaches have limited success, many people remain overweight and must cope with stigma for years.

The workplace is a particular sphere where overweight people may be vulnerable to discriminatory attitudes. A number of studies have investigated weight-based discrimination in employment. The results point to prejudice, insensitivity, and inequity in work settings[106]. The unfair treatment of obese people, especially women, has been found in virtually all stages of employment, including selection, placement, compensation, promotion, discipline and discharge[108]. A longitudinal study by Baum and Ford (2004) suggested that variables such as job discrimination, health-related factors and/or obese workers' behaviour patterns may be channels through which obesity affects wages of both men and women[109].

Effects of negative attitudes among healthcare workers towards obese people

Very negative attitudes about overweight individuals have been reported among doctors, nurses and medical students. Overweight people may be reluctant to seek medical care, especially for their obesity, because they believe that they will be criticised and even humiliated; hence screening and treatment for diseases may be delayed[106]. In a study by Maiman (1979) 87% of healthcare professionals specialising in nutrition believed that obese persons were indulgent; 74% believed that they had family problems, and 32% believed that they lacked will power[110].

Obesity-related stigma and prejudice among children

The strong prejudice against overweight people[104,111] is evident among children[112] including those as young as four years of age. A British study of 180 predominantly lean 4-11 year-olds[113] describes how professionally drawn pictures of fat children, compared with those of

normal and under-weight children, attracted much more negative attributions. Fat children were thought of as ugly, lazy, stupid, and selfish[113]. The fact that children enter adolescence with such clear impressions of the contempt and rejection extended to those who are overweight, provides insight into why body weight concerns wield such a powerful influence during the teenage years.

Obesity related stigma and prejudice among adolescents

A study by Falkner et al (2001) found that obese girls when compared with their average weight counterparts were less likely to hang out with friends, were more likely to report serious emotional problems in the past year, were more likely to report hopelessness, and more likely to report a suicide attempt in the past year[114]. Obese girls were also more likely to report being held back a grade at school. Obese boys were also less likely to hang out with friends, more likely to feel that their friends did not care about them, more likely to report having serious problems in the past year, and more likely to quit school.

Overweight adolescents are less likely to marry when they become adults compared with average weight cohorts, and obese adolescent girls complete less schooling and have lower household incomes as adults than those who are not obese. These social and psychological difficulties associated with obesity may be related to the stigma and prejudice that obese children experience, which hinder their social development during childhood and adolescence[104].

Obese adolescents report experiencing more victimisation than their peers[115]. Obese boys reported being teased, punched, hit, and kicked more than their overweight and average weight peers. Obese girls reported that their classmates refused to spend time with them, gave them the silent treatment, and would not sit near them at class. Because adolescents rely on their peers for the development and maintenance of their self-image, self-acceptance and sense of belonging, the rejection that obese teens experience from their peers can have devastating effects on their social and psychological health[115]. After delivery young adolescent mothers have been shown to reject reliable forms of contraception due to body weight concerns[116].

Coping with stigma

Obesity is linked to a variety of health problems; hence it is critical to prevent additional problems created by stigma.

Obese individuals may deal with stigma related to their condition in a number of ways[107]:

- confirming the negative perceptions ascribed to them by others
- attempting to explain their overweight as resulting for example from events that they could not control, such as medications with side-effects, pressures to eat from family members, or genetics
- directly confronting the 'perpetrator' of stigma
- participation in public groups to protest against weight stigmatisation
- avoidance of social interaction
- attempting to lose weight.

Identification of coping strategies may provide healthcare professionals with tools to help obese clients.

The stigma of overweight limits treatment in several ways: it reduces an individual's confidence about the possibility of change and inappropriately narrows the focus of enquiry to developing ways to deal with the individual as opposed to the environment. **Prejudice against the overweight and obese is maintained because stigma is seen as part of the solution to obesity, when in fact it is part of the problem.** Without changes in societal attitude towards obesity and in the widespread weight prejudice that exists, coping strategies to deal with stigma may have limited success.

THE ECONOMIC PERSPECTIVE

General principles

Obesity is associated with premature death and excess morbidity, and hence has attracted the interest of governments concerned with the welfare of their citizens. Obesity has also attracted the interest of economists, where the issues are consumer sovereignty, externalities, the extent to which economics has any contribution to make in understanding the causal factors behind obesity, and in contributing to policy interventions designed to reduce obesity[117, 118, 119, 120, 121, 122].

As a general rule the presumption is that consumers know what is best for themselves, even if the outcome of their actions may not conform to others' or professionals' beliefs. This presumption lies at the heart of non-intervention by the state in many activities of its citizens, particularly so when it comes to their economic decisions. **In the case of obesity it is argued by some that people who are obese are making a rational choice, in that excess eating and less exercise is viewed as better than the alternative. If, as a result, life is shortened and people suffer various forms of ill-health, that is their choice. However this model may be too simplistic. Throughout this report we show that in fact there are many influences outside individuals' direct control that predispose them to poorer health choices.**

In the last decade increased working hours and increasing congestion, have resulted in much less free time for exercise and meal preparation at home. Consumers would not necessarily be aware of the relationship between calorie intake – established over a long time and changed mainly by reference to convenience foods and eating out – physical work effort, absence of exercise and obesity. This is particularly so since technical obesity is not obviously gross overweight. The issue is compounded when children are considered. It is self-evident that children cannot have all the information necessary to make rational choices, indeed many will not have reached a stage where rationality arises. Some have interpreted this simple fact as evidence that market decisions are inevitably flawed. However it is equally self-evident that decisions must necessarily be made on behalf of children by parents or other adults. There is no reason to believe that parents have not the best interest of their children at heart. Indeed the converse almost certainly applies in the vast majority of families. These factors alone would warrant government intervention in terms of making information available and putting other supportive interventions in place.

Assessment of the impact of overweight and obesity

There must be very few markets where consumers have the information necessary to make optimal decisions. The issue is one of proportionality as a minimum estimate. Is the damage from obesity small? It would be very hard to argue this. **The number of premature deaths annually attributable to obesity is currently approximately 2,000.**[†] There are costs associated with premature death. There is a great deal of confusion about this, as some have valued only the lost production in measuring the cost of premature death. It is very easy to see why this approach is defective, because it places no value on those retired or permanently unemployed. The alternative approach is to obtain the value of a statistical life based on a willingness to pay to avoid death. It is also possible to infer the willingness by society to pay to avoid death from the cost associated with improving roads at danger spots, additional cost arising from increased safety features where society directly undertakes the expenditure. The

[†] Estimate derived from UK figure, National Audit Office (2001)

problem with some of these latter measures is that the differences are very large. Another approach is to measure the value of a life saved from the cost imposed by new regulatory requirements. However the value of life estimated from such work often highlights the political damage caused by some form of death, for example rail accident deaths are accorded more political weight than road traffic deaths. **In spite of this we do have some measures that could be used. At the lower end of the scale is the National Roads Authority estimate for 2002 of a fatal road accident, at €1,357,489[123]. This would place the value of the overall loss of life from obesity at €2.7bn. This is not trivial. The recommended figure to be used in environmental cost benefit analysis in the EU is €1.4m-€2m: so, taking the higher of these figures, the value of the loss of life is placed at €4bn.** These estimates are based on the current level of premature death.

An estimate has been arrived at for the number of children affected by overweight and/or obesity on the island of Ireland. Extrapolating from UK data, this estimate is given as 327,000 overweight and obese children and rising at a rate of 10,750 children per year[124]. Given present levels of obesity among the young it is clear in simple mathematical terms that the numbers dying much earlier than they should will increase dramatically over the next fifty years unless current trends can be changed. Unfortunately time does not permit a demographic/ epidemiological profile to be generated, but it is not difficult to see where the numbers are going.

The government is also concerned about obesity because of the externalities associated with it. The most obvious externality is the healthcare costs arising from obesity, resulting in higher costs than necessary. This affects both tax-driven and insurance-driven healthcare systems. Obesity, the result of private actions by individuals, imposes costs on others through higher taxes, or higher insurance premia, and, given the ever-present waiting list for hospital care, through increased pain and suffering on others arising from delays in treatment. The actual healthcare costs have not been directly estimated, but potential risks have been identified elsewhere in this strategy document. They cover hypertension, type 2 diabetes, excess cholesterol, and stroke among a range of illnesses affecting adults, while among children there may be a slightly different incidence of illness, including asthma, and young adult problems. Obesity may in fact threaten significant gains achieved in cardiovascular health over the last few years. For children some of these problems will remain with them throughout their lives.

The very fact of imposing avoidable costs on others is another reason why government should be interested in preventing obesity. Estimated in-patient costs in 2003 from the Department of Health and Children were given as just over €150,000 where obesity was listed as the primary diagnosis. The proportion of diagnosis attributable to obesity has been estimated as just under €30million (see table 3.1). For England the cost of treating obesity and its consequences was estimated by the Auditor General at £0.5bn in 1998[125]. Determining the true direct healthcare costs for Ireland will prove difficult, because a significant amount of healthcare expenditure is not identified by illness, is privately financed and also, for some, is treated in private institutions. The methodology used in England is instructive, and the numbers derived are the basis of the estimates used here. Obesity was defined as a BMI of 30 or greater in the English study. The approach involved estimating two types of cost: the cost of treating obesity and the costs of treating the consequences of obesity. The direct costs to the health services were defined as the costs to the NHS of treating obesity directly and treating the illnesses associated with it. These were estimated by taking a prevalence-based, costs of illness approach, using actual published primary data for England. Data on the costs of treating illness are available in England.

Table 3.1: Consequences of obesity in all HIPE reporting hospitals

Numbers and costs of inpatient discharges for selected diagnoses and for those estimated as attributable to obesity, 2003.

Principal Diagnosis	Inpatient Discharges			Inpatient Discharges Attributable to Obesity		
	N (a)	Total Cost	Average Case Cost (b)	Estimated %(c)	Estimated N(d)	Estimated Cost(e)
Colon cancer	1,569	€13,351,184	€8,509	29	455	€3,871,844
Rectal cancer	1,579	€11,995,889	€7,597	1	16	€119,959
Endometrial cancer	400	€2,205,491	€5,514	14	56	€308,769
Ovarian cancer	883	€5,764,103	€6,528	13	115	€749,333
Prostate cancer	1,564	€7,387,915	€4,724	3	47	€221,637
Type 2 Diabetes	899	€3,704,530	€4,121	47	423	€1,741,128
Gout	170	€503,320	€2,961	47	80	€236,561
Hypertension	2,297	€7,956,905	€3,464	36	827	€2,864,484
Myocardial Infarction	5,144	€32,446,880	€6,308	18	926	€5,840,435
Angina pectoris	234	€863,362	€3,690	15	35	€129,504
Stroke	9,818	€64,725,802	€6,593	6	589	€3,883,545
Gallstones	6,276	€25,370,991	€4,043	15	941	€3,805,647
Osteoarthritis	5,863	€47,827,280	€8,157	12	704	€5,739,277
Total	**36,696**	**€224,103,651**			**5,213**	**€29,512,123**

(c) National Audit Office (2001). Tackling Obesity in England.

(d) Estimated N = (a)(c)/100.*

(e) Estimated Cost = (b)(d).*

Source: Department of Health and Children and Department of Public Health, Health Services Executive Eastern Region.

Direct healthcare costs

The cost of treating obesity in England was estimated from the costs of GPs, hospital admissions and outpatient attendances, and the cost of drugs prescribed to help people lose weight. The total cost of this was estimated at £9.4 million in 1998, with the bulk of the cost being GP consultations, covering over 500,000 consultations. However the consultation numbers were based on 1991-92 data, and it was believed that the number of consultations had increased significantly from that time. Nevertheless the direct costs of treating obesity were small.

However the costs of treating the consequences of obesity were not small. The methodology here was more complicated: medical literature was examined to determine the proportion of various diseases that was attributable to obesity, based on the relative risk of obese individuals developing the disease compared with the risk for people who were not obese. The basic source of relative risk data was United States data. For each illness the total costs were estimated, taking account of GP consultations, hospital contacts, and cost of prescriptions. The five main diseases, accounting for almost 90% of the total cost, were hypertension, type 2 diabetes, angina pectoris, heart attack and osteoarthritis. The biggest cost was the cost of prescriptions, followed by hospital contacts. The overall cost was estimated at £469.9 million. Table 3.2, adapted from the Auditor General's report is instructive.

Table 3.2: The costs of treating the consequences of obesity in England in 1998

	Attributable cases (% of total cases)	Cost of GP consultations £m	Cost of hospital contacts £m	Cost of prescriptions £m	Total cost £m
Hypertension	794,276 (36)	25.5	7.7	101.6	134.8
Type 2 diabetes	270,504 (47)	7.9	36.7	78.9	123.5
Angina pectoris	90,776 (15)	2.8	35.3	46.6	84.7
Myocardial infarction	28,027 (18)	0.6	41.6	0	42.2
Osteoarthritis	194,683 (12)	4.7	14.5	15.6	34.8
Others		3.4	41.9	4.6	49.9
Total		**44.9**	**177.7**	**247.3**	**469.9**

Source: National Audit Office, 2001

Taken together the direct costs are just under £470 million. While this estimate seems low, the general methodology is sound, and what seems to be driving down the costs is the low cost of provision of services. The average GP cost in the relevant time period was £13 per consultation, which seems low compared with costs in Ireland at the same time, and drug expenditure is influenced by the role of pharmacies in the UK, which has the effect of minimising drug costs. **On a pro-rata population basis, allowing for differences in the cost of drugs, GP visits, and hospital costs, this puts the cost in Ireland in 2002 at some €70 million.** This is an order of magnitude only, and more precise costs would require a great deal of primary research. While on the face of it this seems a relatively low number it is more than twice that estimated for the healthcare costs of environmental tobacco smoke, which places it in context.

Indirect costs

There are also indirect costs associated with obesity. These include workplace costs: days lost due to illness arising from obesity, and for those who are obese possibly lower wages because of discrimination arising from their obesity. Finally there are output losses due to output foregone as a result of premature death. We have no reasonable estimates of this. For England, the Auditor General estimated the total indirect costs at £2.6 billion in 1998[125]. On a pro-rata basis, and allowing for increased costs since, this would place the indirect costs at some €0.37 billion. Together the direct and indirect costs are about €0.4 billion.

It has to be said that these costs are swamped by the values obtained by considering lives lost. There is a danger that looking only at the public finance cost or the output lost will obscure the fundamental point that the real loss is the premature death. With road traffic deaths this point is well recognised by the society at large, because the concern is with the loss of life, rather than the loss of output.

It also must be stressed that these numbers are based on the estimated current situation. A continuation of the present trends in relation to obesity, particularly in children, will lead to rapidly escalating numbers of obese persons, and rapidly accelerating direct costs, indirect costs, and loss of life. This 'steady state' situation needs to be explored more fully because the issue is not just the costs estimated here.

The cost of physical inactivity

There are serious economic consequences associated with the obesity epidemic and physical inactivity. The current CMO report in the UK estimated the cost of physical inactivity at £8.2 billion annually. This figure includes both the cost of the NHS and the cost to the economy such as days lost from work[126].

The healthcare costs associated with obesity in the United States were estimated at over 75 billion dollars in 2000, costs associated with physical inactivity were estimated to be another 24 billion dollars. The costs related to inactivity and obesity alone account for approximately 9.4% of the national health expenditure in the United States[127]. In Canada physical inactivity accounts for about 6% of national health care expenditure[127].

The contribution of economics

The final issue to be considered is the input that economics can make to the solution of the problem of obesity. First the causal factors must be identified. Research elsewhere suggests that the decline in food prices relative to the price of other goods encourages excess eating. This decline itself reflects the great technological changes that have taken place in food production in the past half century, driven in part by bizarre pricing as in the case of CAP, where prices were above the market clearing level for decades, encouraged excess production and dumping of agricultural products on world markets, while attempting to maintain high prices to consumers in the EU and huge subsidies, as in the case of US agriculture. Ex-farm prices in the EU are now in decline because of necessary changes to CAP, and food prices to consumers are increasing less than the general price index, effectively making food better value relative to other products. Over the period 2000 to 2004 food prices in Ireland increased by 11.4% while overall prices increased by 16% – in 2004 food prices actually fell by 0.3% while overall prices increased by 2.2%. These relative price shifts encourage food consumption. In the case of the US the big increase in food output did lead directly to reduced food prices[128].

In the case of Ireland most foods are VAT free, keeping prices lower than otherwise would be the case, and this encourages increased consumption. In the case of eating out VAT is paid, but at below the standard rate and this is reflected in relatively good value for food where commodity service (as in the case of many fast-food outlets) is the norm, compared with expenditure on other goods. There is a very big difference in price and in changes in price between commodity service restaurants and service intensive restaurants. The latter have much higher prices and have experienced substantial increases in prices in recent years driven by increased labour costs, while in the former prices have not increased so rapidly, thus making them relatively cheaper.

The reasons for this derived from concerns with the ability of those on low incomes to afford food, given the relatively high proportion of food in their expenditure. This proportion has changed dramatically over the past two decades. **The current pattern of food purchasing by vulnerable groups is reflected in the accessibility of cheaper, convenient food that does not comply with dietary recommendations**[129,130]. Furthermore low food prices benefit all, not just the poor. A more rational approach would be to have similar VAT rates across all household expenditure, with greater income support for those on lower incomes, financed by the increased VAT receipts. If relative prices are different, then people will make different choices in relation to food and other expenditure. This would also affect the other main characteristics of increased food consumption, that is to say the increase in the use of convenience foods and low-cost restaurants.

It is not just a question of the cost relative to other goods. The past two decades have been characterised by big changes in the workplace, manifested in increased participation by both partners in households. This has occurred simultaneously with increased working hours, mostly informally undertaken, and perhaps not officially measured. At the same time increased congestion and consequent increased travel times have limited the time people have for other activities, including exercise, preparing meals at home, and even taking time to buy the materials for preparing meals at home. The scarce commodity is time.

There is some evidence from the United States that the time constraint is very important in relation to child obesity, where the longer the working hours of the mother the greater the risk of obesity in children, but this factor explains only a very small proportion of the increase in obesity and is likely to be confounded by other economic factors, including the necessity to work by women in poorer economic circumstances[117]. Of course this reflects very traditional patterns of the distribution of household activities between partners, and there may be some change in this, as many other traditional practices die out. It is unrealistic to think that dual working households with children will revert to single working parent households, particularly as policy in Ireland, reinforced in the recent budget with the extension of individualisation, is geared towards increasing participation of both spouses. Increasing obesity among children may be a consequence of this and it remains a matter of concern that insufficient thought was given to this issue.

The congestion problem caused by increasing urbanisation can be eased, and on completion of existing infrastructure projects the situation will improve. The National Spatial Strategy, and the planning guidelines evolved from this, will fundamentally alter the new distribution of housing, its density and travel patterns. This must be supported by improved public transport, as many local authorities charged with implementing the planning guidelines have argued, and it must be supported by congestion pricing to change behaviour. Otherwise the congestion will simply get worse.

There are other things government can do. There is some evidence, based on data on women's health, that having a Leaving Certificate is associated with a lower BMI. This suggests that a solid education in itself is empowering to women, for themselves and as caregivers to their families, and re-enforces the key role played by equitable public policy generally in reducing social inequalities[131]. More information targeted on likely affected groups may be desirable, and more direct interventions through the administrative system may be called for, covering food standards, requirements on the availability of different forms of food etc designed to change eating patterns. It is an observable fact that access to food more consistent with avoiding obesity is poorer in low income areas than in high income areas. This reflects the market as perceived by suppliers, because the same companies will be offering a different range of products in different markets. If information were widely available and absorbed then changes in consumption patterns would induce changes in supplies. It is not clear that changes in supply availability undertaken on its own would be successful, unless all suppliers acted in concert, and there is the potential for losses if consumers do not respond. Direct commodity subsidies are unlikely to be successful, because they cannot be limited to target groups, so possibly the only mechanism would be supplier subsidies to cover additional costs. Even with this there are moral hazard issues unless such subsidies are capped.

Finally, it is worth noting that obesity occurs because calorie intake exceeds calorie consumption, and calorie expenditure has decreased over the past half century. Most of the emphasis has been on factors that encourage calorie intake, but a big change has been in the area of calorie expenditure as manual work has been replaced by machine work. People are not having enough physical exercise in their workplace. Again this is a function of information, where the importance of exercise needs to be stressed, and opportunity, where people have facilities for exercising. There is no singular approach to this that government can adopt, it needs to proceed on all fronts: swimming pools, keep fit establishments, access to walking areas, safe public parks, elimination of restrictions on using green areas in estates for exercise, and so on.

THE HEALTH IMPACT OF OBESITY

The World Health Organisation estimated that about half a million people in North America and Europe died from obesity related diseases in 2002 and this is set to increase by one third over the next twenty years if nothing is done[18].

In England it has been estimated by the National Audit Office that obesity is responsible for more than 9,000 premature deaths each year and reduces life expectancy on average by nine years[125]. Cases of type 2 diabetes are starting to emerge in childhood with the first cases being diagnosed in children in England in 2002.

The health consequences of obesity range from a number of non-fatal complaints that impact on the quality of life – such as respiratory difficulties, musclo-skeletal problems, skin problems and infertility – to complaints that increase the risk of premature death including non-insulin dependent diabetes, gall-bladder disease, cancers and cardiovascular problems (hypertension, stroke and coronary heart disease).

Overweight and obese individuals (BMI of 25 and above) are at an increased risk of

- premature death
- type 2 (non-insulin dependent) diabetes, insulin resistance, glucose intolerance, hyperinsulinemia
- hypertension
- dyslipidemia, high blood cholesterol
- coronary heart disease, angina pectoris
- congestive heart failure
- stroke
- gallstones, cholescystitis and cholelithiasis
- gout
- osteoarthritis
- obstructive sleep apnoea and respiratory problems
- some types of cancer (such as endometrial, breast, prostate, and colon)
- complications of pregnancy
- poor female reproductive health (such as menstrual irregularities, infertility, irregular ovulation)
- bladder control problems (such as stress incontinence)
- uric acid nephrolithiasis or kidney stones
- psychological disorders (such as depression, eating disorders, distorted body image, and low self-esteem).

Diabetes mellitus

Diabetes mellitus can be divided into different types depending on the underlying pathological mechanisms. Type 2 diabetes has been associated with onset in older people usually resulting from insulin resistance, which is a state in which normal concentrations of insulin produce a subnormal biological response. It is recognised that obesity is a major modifiable risk factor for type 2 diabetes. In the UK 75% of adults with newly diagnosed type 2 diabetes are overweight or obese[132]. Historically type 2 diabetes has been associated with adults and older people but with overweight and obesity increasingly affecting children more and more children are being diagnosed with this type of diabetes. Obesity can reduce the life expectancy of people with type 2 diabetes by up to eight years[133]. Patients with diabetes mellitus have a twofold to fourfold increased risk of developing cerebrovascular (stroke), coronary and peripheral vascular disease than those who do not.

Several studies have shown the increased risk of developing diabetes mellitus as weight increases. In particular abdominal obesity has been shown to be a major risk factor for type 2 diabetes. The relative risk of diabetes increases by 25% for each additional unit of BMI over 22kg/m^2.

Reducing insulin resistance is important in managing non-insulin dependent diabetes, for example by losing weight and by aerobic exercise. **It is estimated that at least half of all cases of type 2 diabetes would be eliminated if weight gain in adults could be prevented.**

Hypertension

Studies show that the prevalence of high blood pressure increases progressively with higher levels of BMI in men and women. (High blood pressure is defined as mean systolic blood pressure >= 140 mmHg or mean systolic blood pressure = 90 mmHg or currently taking anti-hypertension medication). The relative risk of high blood pressure if BMI is greater or equal to 30 compared to less than 25 is 2.1 for men and 1.9 for women[134].

The direct or indirect association between blood pressure and weight or BMI has been shown by a number of studies. A 10 kg higher body weight has been associated with a 3.0 mmHg higher systolic and a 2.3 mmHg higher diastolic blood pressure. Obesity and hypertension are co-morbidity risk factors for the development of cardiovascular disease.

Coronary heart disease

Studies indicate that overweight, obesity and excess abdominal fat are related to important coronary heart disease (CHD) risk factors including high levels of total cholesterol, LDL cholesterol, triglycerides, blood pressure, fibrinogen and insulin and low levels of HDL-cholesterol. They are also associated with increased morbidity and mortality from coronary heart disease including angina pectoris.

Dyslipidaemia

A BMI greater than 25 is associated with higher total cholesterol levels, higher triglyceride and LDL-cholesterol levels and lower HDL-cholesterol levels. The link between total serum cholesterol and coronary heart disease is largely due to low-density lipoprotein (LDL). This lipoprotein is the predominant atherogenic lipoprotein and therefore the primary target of

cholesterol lowering therapy. Data suggests that a 10mg/dl rise in LDL-cholesterol corresponds to an approximate 10% increase in coronary heart disease over a 5-10 year period[134]. A 1% reduction in LDL levels is associated with a 2% reduction in coronary heart disease and a 1% increase in HDL levels is associated with a 3% reduction in coronary heart disease death[135,136].

Congestive Heart failure

Overweight and obesity have been identified as independent risk factors for congestive heart failure (CHF) in a number of studies including the Framington Heart Study. Obesity can result in alteration in the cardiac structure and function, which can lead to congestive heart failure.

Stroke

Studies show a relationship between ischaemic but not haemorrhagic strokes and therefore in studies of fatal outcomes of strokes only a weak relationship between strokes and overweight has been demonstrated.

Gallstones

The risk of gallstones increases with adult weight, especially in women.

Osteoarthritis

The risk of developing osteoarthritis increases with overweight and this association is stronger in women. An increase in weight is also associated with increased pain in osteoarithic weight bearing joints. Weight loss has been shown to improve pain free movement and leads to a reduction in the use of pain relief.

Obstructive sleep apnoea

Sleep apnoea obesity hyperventilation syndrome occurs in 5% of severely obese individuals and is potentially a life-threatening syndrome. It is found in relation to upper body obesity in particular. Obstructive sleep apnoea can induce extreme hypoxaemia and this can lead to cardiac failure.

Cancer

Breast cancer

There is evidence that obesity is associated with a twofold increase in the risk of breast cancer in postmenopausal women whereas among pre-menopausal women it is associated with a reduced incidence[137]. The major risk factor for post-menopausal breast cancer is oestrogen and the main source of this in these women is in peripheral fat. **There is evidence that even a modest weight gain increases the risk of postmenopausal breast cancer.** The effect of increased body mass on breast cancer risk seems to vary according to timing of obesity onset and its persistence into adulthood. The USA Nurses Health Study provided evidence that the timing of weight gain is important[138]. Obesity manifesting in the teenage years is associated with a reduced risk of breast cancer before, and less so after, the menopause; while the development of obesity after the age of eighteen years was related to a higher risk of postmenopausal but not premenopausal breast cancer risk[138]. The mechanisms whereby obesity during adolescence is associated with a reduced breast cancer risk are uncertain but likely to include the anovulatory cycles associated with adolescent obesity[139].

Endometrial cancer
Although endometrial cancer is not as common as breast cancer the risk is increased by obesity.
Colon cancer
A number of studies have shown a relationship between obesity and colon cancer in men but a weaker association in women.

Women's reproductive health

Obesity can lead to menstrual irregularity and increases the risk of infertility.

Pregnancy
Pregnancy can result in weight gain and retention of this weight, with over 40% in one study reporting that they retained 4kg(9lb) of their gained weight after pregnancy. **Obesity during pregnancy is associated with increased morbidity for both mother and child.** This includes hypertension, gestational diabetes, difficulties in labour and delivery, higher risks with anaesthesia, congenital malformations, and in particular neural tube defects. However a certain amount of weight gain is desirable in pregnancy and therefore a balance should be sought for the optimum weight gain for each woman during pregnancy. It is recommended that all pregnant women should have a BMI recorded and measured at the beginning of pregnancy. Studies show that very overweight women would benefit from a reduced weight gain during pregnancy to help reduce the risk to the infant.

Psychological effects of obesity

Obesity has also been linked to several adverse psychological states, among which is low self-esteem[140]. This negative psychological effect is assumed to be due to the social stigma attached to obesity in Western society. A United States study[141] found that adiposity had a negative effect on the level of self-esteem in girls as young as nine to ten years, and that there were racial differences in the psychological impact of obesity. Certain psychological problems, including binge eating disorder and depression are more common among obese persons than they are in the general population[142].

Obese individuals may suffer from social stigmatisation and discrimination, and severely obese people may experience greater risk of impaired psychosocial and physical functioning causing a negative impact on their quality of life. **The stigma of overweight is based on the erroneous notion that people are entirely responsible (and therefore to blame) for their own weight. Obese people internalise this view and subsequently blame themselves for the negative attitudes of others towards them[106]. The socially ascribed 'overweight woman' is stigmatised and encouraged to monitor herself in a never ending process of self surveillance to conform to a culturally acceptable body image[143].**

Depression

Studies carried out by both Carpenter (2000) and Istvan (1992) reported that obese women were more likely to be depressed than average weight peers; the reverse was found for men (obese men are less likely to report a history of depression than average weight men)[144, 145]. Data from the third national Health and Nutrition Examination Survey (1998-1994) were used to examine the relationship between obesity and depression. Onyike et al (2003) found that obesity is associated with depression mainly among persons with severe obesity[146]. Investigations of the relationship between quality of life and level of BMI have reported that quality of life impairment worsens with increasing obesity. The question of whether obesity precedes depression or whether an existing mood disturbance predisposes to increased weight has been examined and it has been suggested that depression precedes obesity in adolescent girls but not boys and that obesity precedes depression in older adults[105].

Health impact of obesity in childhood

The immediate and short term problems that overweight and obese children may experience include type 2 diabetes, respiratory, cardiovascular and orthopaedic problems, social isolation and psychological effects. **The prevalence of type 2 diabetes in children and adolescents has increased in recent years and this appears to be associated with the increasing levels of overweight and obesity in children.** The most important long-term consequence of childhood obesity is its persistence into adulthood with many studies showing that BMI in childhood is significantly related to BMI in adulthood. Childhood obesity is predictive of adult risk factors and morbidity for coronary heart disease. There are very few long-term studies available to indicate whether childhood obesity is independently related to coronary heart disease in adulthood or whether the increased risk associated with childhood obesity is mediated by adult weight status. However, there seems to be an independent risk associated with obesity during male adolescence. The Harvard Growth Study showed an increased mortality risk associated with overweight during male adolescence, which persisted even among those who lost weight and were lean during adulthood[147].

Overweight children have been found to be more likely to be involved in bullying than their peers. It has been found that overweight children are more likely than their peers to be victims and in some case perpetrators of teasing, name calling and physical bullying[148].

Benefits of weight loss

Weight loss in overweight and obese individuals improves physical, metabolic and endrocrinological complications. It can also improve depression, anxiety, psychosocial functioning, mood and the quality of life. For those that are already obese even a modest weight loss can have substantial benefits. A 10 kg loss is associated with a 20% fall in total mortality and a 10% reduction in total cholesterol. Further studies show that intentional weight loss in overweight women of 0.5-9 kg can lead to a 20% fall in total mortality, a 40-50% reduction in mortality in obesity related cancers and a 30-40% reduction in diabetes related deaths[134].

Physical inactivity: *the risks to health*

Physical inactivity and obesity are related to many chronic diseases and considered to be a serious and growing public health concern[149]. There is substantial evidence that demonstrates that inactive lifestyles have a negative effect on both individual and public health. The World Health Organisation estimated that physical inactivity causes approximately 2 million deaths each year with the global prevalence of 17%[127].

The health risks associated with being physically inactive include obesity, type 2 diabetes, cardiovascular disease, hypertension, osteoporosis, colon cancer and premature mortality[150]. Physical inactivity plays a role in coronary heart disease and the continued prevalence of physical inactivity is a threat to the progress in reduction of mortality associated with many chronic diseases including CHD [149].

Physical fitness is a potential predictor of all-cause and cardiovascular mortality. In a study on >25,000 males, having a low level of physical fitness conferred the same risk of all-cause mortality as smoking or hypertension in normal weight and overweight subjects[151]. In obese males, physical fitness was a better predictor of all-cause mortality and had a similar risk to those with a previous heart attack or stroke.

Physical inactivity is a serious concern with regard to children and adolescents, because habits established in childhood may continue to adulthood[152]. Although physical inactivity alone does not cause obesity, there is a relationship between sedentary lifestyles and prevalence of overweight and obesity[152]. Monitoring physical activity levels in adolescence is critical because of its importance in preventing the onset of obesity and obesity-related illness later in life[41].

Physical activity: *the benefits to health*

Physical activity plays a vital role in our health and well-being and is considered to be a key factor in the prevention of overweight and obesity[149]. Regular physical activity has been shown to reduce the morbidity and mortality related to many chronic diseases[153] and epidemiological studies show that overweight and obese persons who are currently engaged in physical activity show a smaller risk of weight gain[42].

The recent United States Surgeon General's report concluded that physiological effects from physical activity included benefits to the cardiovascular and musculo-skeletal systems, with benefits to the metabolic, endocrine, and immune systems. It has been shown that individuals who have high levels of physical activity have a lower mortality rate than those with sedentary lifestyles[149] There is substantial evidence that physical activity can be protective against many degenerative diseases and is a significant modifier of morbidity and mortality associated with overweight and obesity[86]. Physical activity benefits all individuals regardless of body composition and recent findings suggest that overweight and obese individuals can experience the same health benefits as lean individuals.

Physical activity plays an important role in cardiovascular health, has been found to lower blood pressure and can help prevent cardiovascular disease[153]. Such activity brings an important reduction in risk of mortality and morbidity for those overweight and obese. The United States Surgeon General's report found strong support for the protective effect of physical activity on the development of type 2 diabetes[149]. Body weight and physical inactivity together are estimated to account for up to one-third of the most common cancers, including breast (postmenopausal), kidney, colon, endometrium and oesophagus[153].

According to the Chief Medical Officer's report from the UK adults who are physically active have a 20-30% reduced risk of premature death and a 50% reduced risk of developing major chronic diseases such as coronary heart disease, stroke, diabetes and cancers[126]. Physically active individuals have less GP visits, fewer days in hospital and require less medication per annum than physically inactive individuals. In addition to the physical health benefits there are important mental health benefits such as improved mood, a sense of achievement, relaxation and decrease in stress that can result from regular physical activity[126].

4 The CHALLENGE for SOCIETY

4 The CHALLENGE for SOCIETY

The obesity-promoting environment has become known as the 'obesogenic' environment[154]. This term has emerged as a means of encapsulating changing lifestyles in the late twentieth and early twenty-first centuries. In a world dominated by sedentary pursuits and convenience foods, health experts are increasingly concerned about weight problems in young people particularly. The term 'obesogenic' is a product of such concerns, as individuals attempt to describe the social factors which have contributed to this public health issue[155].

As is shown in this report, the obesogenic environment is progressively reinforced by many cultural changes that make the adoption of healthier lifestyles, especially for children and adolescents, more and more difficult. The environmental influences on the amount and type of food eaten and the amount and type of physical activity taken are many and significant. For example physical environment influences include on the one hand food and drinks industry production, retail and supply policies and, on the other hand, the availability of cycle ways, safe streets and good public transport. The economic environment influences include food taxes and subsidies, food prices, the cost of cycleways, the cost of school sport and the cost of gym fees. The socio-cultural environment influences include consumer demand, family-eating patterns, pressure from food advertising, attitudes to recreation, and concerns for safety among schools' authorities. At the centre of these changing environments is the adult or child who requires certain skills to enable him or her to make 'healthy' choices for life.

The energy balance

Energy intake is just one side of the weight equation with adequate energy expenditure or physical activity being essential to maintain balance. There is ample evidence that rates of 'passive exercise' – physical activity undertaken as part of everyday life – have declined (see Chapter 2). Twentieth-century labour-saving devices, from cars to e-mail, are ubiquitous and have reduced energy needs, as has the shift of a large proportion of the workforce from manual labour to white-collar jobs that require little activity. There is less routine travel by foot or bicycle and the physical elements of housework, shopping and other necessary activities have decreased. This affects both adults and children: children are driven to school and spend more time watching television. Other elements of modern civilisation, such as central heating, lessen the cost of maintaining body temperature. Dangerous neighbourhoods discourage people from walking dogs, pushing buggies, playing football, jogging, or permitting children to play outdoors. Many rural and suburban neighbourhoods are structured for the convenience of car drivers; they may not have footpaths and may lack local shops, social outlets or other facilities within walking distance.

The school environment provides an opportunity to reach almost all children in the first two decades of their lives and thus is an ideal setting in which to practice health promoting behaviour such as healthy eating and physical activity. However competing academic priorities have forced some schools to relegate physical education to the status of a 'non-essential' subject. One Irish study for example found only a single school in Limerick that met the Department of Education and Science guidelines of 120 minutes of physical education at Junior and Senior cycle[156]. Added to this is the fact that facilities for physical education in some schools are often inadequate.

Influences on physical activity

There are many factors that influence an individual's level of physical activity including demographic, social, cultural and environmental variables [157]. In the adult population factors associated with age, lifestyle, work and the proximity of facilities are often indicated as causes of low levels of physical activity. The decline of work-related physical activity, reduced activity for daily living and increased sedentary behaviour are all factors that contribute to low energy expenditure [82].

The social determinants of physical activity include factors such as socio-economic status, education level, gender, family and peer group influences[150]. They also include personal issues such as perceptions of the benefits of physical activity and attitudes toward physical activity[157]. **In industrialised countries children from lower socio-economic groups have a greater risk of obesity than those from higher socio-economic groups. The reasons for this may not be straightforward but low self-esteem and feelings of disempowerment may be key influences in the high rates of obesity among these socio-economic groups[124].**

The Surgeon General in the United States lists certain factors that influence **adolescent** physical activity[149,180]:

- self-efficacy – the confidence in one's ability to engage in physical activity
- social influences such as parental or peer engagement
- exercise enjoyment
- positive attitudes towards physical education
- lack of sufficient sports facilities[153].

A recent study found that obese children had low levels of physical activity compared to non-obese children of the same age group[158]. The main findings reported that obese children had lower levels of physical activity self-efficacy, were less involved in community-based physical activity organisations and were less likely to have physically active parents. In this study parental physical activity was a strong predictor of physical activity during childhood.

Gender is also an important factor in relation to adolescent physical activity, and must be addressed. It has been found that girls' participation in physical activity is lower than that of boys and is characterised by a sharp decline in adolescence[152, 28]. The low level of participation in physical activity among young girls has implications for both health promotion and school policy. The behaviour patterns established during this period have long-term public health implications[159].

The Surgeon General has also described factors that influence **adult** physical activity in the United States[149,180]:

- self efficacy – the confidence in one's ability to engage in physical activity
- beliefs about the outcome of physical activity
- exercise enjoyment
- social support networks – having friends who engage in physical activity[160]
- availability and proximity of community facilities[153]
- environments conducive to physical activity[153]

The environmental factors have been the least studied in terms of physical activity but are important in determining the potential predictors of physical activity. The geographic location and time of year have been identified as strong predictors of levels of physical activity engagement[161]. Other predictive environmental factors include proximity of facilities, open spaces, parks and safe areas generally[157].

The physical environment of cities and towns impacts on the levels of physical activity undertaken by the population. There is now more of an emphasis on planning communities and transportation systems that promote active transportation[162]. Public transport plays a part in encouraging physical activity because a journey by public transport usually requires walking to get to the end destination, an average walk of about ten minutes in New Zealand by all accounts[163]. The promotion of physical activity through commuting encourages the greater use of public transport and therefore supports the strategies of urban planners and transportation agencies.

Reasons proposed for a decline in walking and cycling include the increasing distances needed for typical everyday activities, increased car ownership and increased volumes of traffic. Suggestions for tackling these factors include traffic calming measures, enhancing footpaths, cycle racks and pressing local authorities to produce local transport plans that will encourage walking and cycling.

If there were a widespread modal shift from the motor vehicle to walking or cycling the health benefits would include reductions in pollution, noise and road traffic injury rates, as well as the potential for increased physical activity. It has been found that low levels of cycling, especially in cities, often correlate with cultures that do not support cycling and with policies that do not plan for the needs of cyclists and pedestrians, particularly safety needs. In countries such as the Netherlands there is a culture of cycling and urban roads and paths are designed to facilitate cycling and walking[86]. Clearly there is a public health imperative to evaluate the effect of all environmental policies and their associations with active transport, recreational physical activity and total physical activity[162].

Changing diets

General dietary recommendations to reduce calorie consumption may not have sufficient impact on the general population[51]. In Ireland lifestyles have changed: jobs are increasingly sedentary and involve longer working hours and longer commuting times. Eating habits have changed from the traditional three meals a day to increasingly continuous eating. This means that people rely more and more on convenience foods, snacking and eating out. Commercial interests have progressively supplied food that is more completely prepared. Eating opportunities surround the public, and peoples' diet choices and consumption are strongly influenced by commercial and business strategies. Collectively, the food and drinks industry – retail, restaurants, manufacturing, processing – creates a strong environmental force encouraging the population's food consumption. Therefore the support of the food and drinks industry is an essential element in changing the population's dietary habits in the direction of healthy eating guidelines. Eating food outside of the home, in cafes and fast-food outlets, has also become more common[16] (see Chapter 2). Facilitating change towards healthier food options in these circumstances needs concerted consumer demand for such options being met by the food industry.

Influences on diet

The amount and type of food we consume is influenced by a range of internal and external cues. Our diet is determined, most importantly, by the availability of food. Our food choice is influenced by liking the taste of particular foods. However, this is only one component in the overall variation in food choice and eating behaviours[164]. **It is generally accepted that in developed countries the main barriers to healthy food choices are access to healthy foodstuffs, their affordability and one's level of disposable income.**

Households with low incomes spend a greater proportion of income on food but in real terms spend less than those on higher incomes. In Ireland those in the bottom 20% of income distribution still spend over 40% of their disposable income on food as against the average percentage spend on food by households, which has decreased from 38% to 20%. Social welfare payments are the main source of income for many low-income groups and therefore are important in determining the living standards of households in these groups. **In Ireland it was found, as it was in the UK, that the foods recommended in the Irish healthy eating dietary guidelines were often more expensive than the less-healthy options[130].** The most common type of retail outlet used by the lower income groups is that of local convenience outlets followed by the local independent traders. Large retail outlets can have a greater choice of healthy affordable food, but may be difficult to access, especially if there is not adequate public transport. The outlets where socially disadvantaged people shopped were less likely to carry a good range of healthy foods and when they did they were more expensive. Research has found for low income groups there are big discrepancies between the amount of money they would need to spend in order to purchase a healthy diet, the amount of money they have available to spend and the amount of money they are currently spending[130].

Access to cooking facilities and the ability to prepare food also influences the type of food consumed. The handing-on of cooking skills through the family is disappearing, experience in the preparation of foods from basic ingredients is no longer widespread. In a study carried out by the National Food Alliance/MORI in 1993, young people were asked: 'Which of these things can you do yourself?'. Ninety-three percent could play computer games, 77% could use a music centre or CD, 61% could programme a video recording, 60% could heat a pizza in the microwave, 54% could make a cake and 38% could cook a jacket potato in the oven[165]. As children become adults and leave home their cooking skills may soon encompass only foods that are convenient and easy to prepare. These foods tend to be high in fat, salt and sugar. Food skills such as handling, hygiene, shopping and storage should be identified and promoted as life skills which are essential in influencing dietary behaviour[166].

Eating family meals can have a healthy influence over diet, particularly in adolescence[226]. A recent study of Irish parents reported that 71% of families normally ate breakfast as a family on weekdays[101]. This percentage was lower (57%) in families with a child who was reported as overweight. Most families in the study reported eating their evening meals together but 36% routinely had their evening meals in front of the TV (45% at weekends).

Food labelling and promotion

Product and food labelling is an essential component of consumer choice. There has been an increase in the number of Irish people reading food labels from 56% in 1998 to 66% in 2002 and they tend to look for ingredient and nutrient information[47]. Research has shown that labels are often confusing, particularly food labelling which prevents the consumer from making an informed purchasing decision[167]. The WHO Global Strategy on Diet, Physical Activity and Health 2004 recommends that consumers should have accurate, standardised and comprehensive information on the content of food items in order to make healthy choices.

The media is one of the most popular vehicles through which consumers receive information and is powerful in influencing food selection and health behaviours[168]. Advertising and marketing practices are designed to increase sales. In Ireland, the 2003 estimates for advertising expenditure on food and beverages were over €132 million[169]. Foods that are high in fat, sugar and salt attracted most of the spend on advertising and this is reflected in their high sales[170]. The International Association of Consumer Food Organisations has highlighted the types of food which are advertised the most compared to the recommended dietary guidelines (Figure 4.1) [171].

Figure 4.1: Proportion of the types of foods advertised in relation to the Food Pyramid

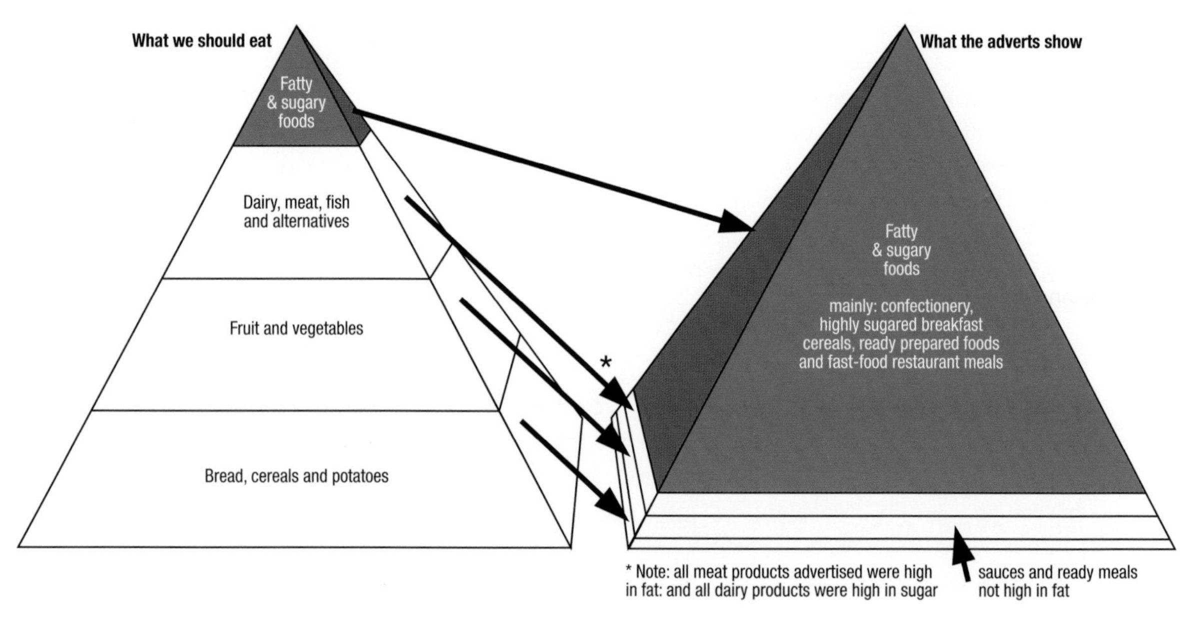

Source: Food Commission, UK, 2003

Promotion of food products takes cognisance of the fact that children are attracted by foods in bright packaging and those accompanied by free gifts or promoted by cartoon characters[172]. Processed foods like chocolates, crisps, soft drinks, pre-sugared breakfast cereals and fast-food meals that are high in salt, sugar or fat are among the most heavily promoted especially by television but these are usually the ones that dietary guidelines emphasise should be eaten the least. Young children are often the target group for the advertising of these products for the simple reason that they have a significant influence on foods bought by parents[173]. A report from the World Health Organisation and the Food and Agriculture Organisation of the United Nations (2003) concluded that the aggressive marketing of these types of food and drinks to young children could increase their risk of becoming obese[42]. 'Part of the consistent, strong relationships between television viewing and obesity in children may relate to the food advertising to which they are exposed[174]'.

Studies on the behavioural effects of advertising find that television has a major influence on the products children ask for and that increased television viewing leads to increased requests for advertised products[175]. Television advertising can create misperceptions among children about the nutritional values of foods and the pursuit of positive health[176]. Many young children, especially those under the age of six, have difficulty understanding that advertising is a tool used to sell products; it is not until children approach the age of twelve that most are able to comprehend the purpose of advertising[177].

Advertising of foods, which affect oral health, was examined by Chestnutt and Ashraf (2002)[225]. During children's TV, 62.5% of advertising time was devoted to foodstuffs, significantly greater than the 18.4% of time spent advertising foods during primetime. Of the time spent advertising foods, during children's TV 73.4% was devoted to products deemed potentially detrimental to oral health (primarily high in sugar), compared to 18.6% similarly categorised during evening television.

A recent Irish study reported that 75% of parents of 7-8 year-olds considered that TV food advertising to children usually promotes 'unhealthy'† foods (SHB, 2004)[101]. In the same survey 50% of parents felt that their children (in first class at school) pressurised them, as a direct result of TV advertisements, to buy certain foods or drinks. The recent Code of Practice launched by the Broadcasting Commission of Ireland takes some steps to address the issue of advertising directed at children on Irish television[99]. Such advertising is not limited just to television. It extends to a broad range of media which are also influential. The power of advertising in the media can be harnessed conversely of course to promote a healthy, balanced lifestyle.

According to a report from the British Food Standards Agency (Hastings, 2003), food promotion does affect children's food preferences, purchasing and consumption behaviour, rather than merely causing brand switching[172]. The literature suggests that food promotion can influence the diet in a variety of ways. However, this does not amount to proof – 'incontrovertible proof simply isn't attainable' [172].

† 'unhealthy' food, defined in this survey as food with a high fat, high salt, high sugar content.

BEST PRACTICE INTERVENTIONS

Policies

Despite considerable rhetoric to the contrary few regions or countries have put in place readily evaluable concerted policy initiatives in relation to obesity. Health education campaigns must be backed by supportive public policy if the weight of evidence on the determinants is correct. The United States, for instance, has delivered a variety of public health campaigns aimed at encouraging healthy eating and physical activity. However, research has shown that 78% of Americans do not believe that their body weight is a serious health concern, although two-thirds of respondents were in fact overweight or obese[178]. This health issue, therefore requires more than health education messages. Nutrition related policies, for instance, have generally focused on providing information such as labelling of food or dietary guidelines. While these are important elements of a healthy policy the discussion must be extended to consider the important role that supply-side public policies play in our food chain, from farm to fork. Agricultural, industrial and economic policies are significant in determining the nature of food available and the environmental conditions under which it is presented[179]. **Fundamental policy change at government level is required to develop a society which can enable people to eat healthily and partake in physical activity.** However such far-reaching change requires direction and monitoring of progress from a lead group or agency to ensure it is fully realised[180] (see Recommendations in Chapter 5).

Prior to the establishment of the National Taskforce on Obesity a review of the role of public policies, the development of relevant industries under these policies, and the contribution these policies may be making as a major environmental factor contributing to the growing obesity problem had not been carried out in Ireland. From a historical perspective public policies initially implemented with valid objectives can, at a later stage, undercut new policies with different and frequently opposing objectives. Established economic, environmental and agricultural policies can serve as formidable impediments to the success of new healthy public policies that are needed to address obesity. Ireland has an important advocacy role to play in addressing these policy issues both at a national and European level (see Recommendations in Chapter 5).

Fiscal policies such as taxing so-called unhealthy foods, and the provision of incentives to encourage the supply of healthy food or access to physical activity have been suggested as a way in which government could intervene to help reverse the trend in obesity[181]. It has been argued that these measures could have the advantage of raising revenue which the government could use to finance other measures to combat obesity such as education programmes or subsidising resources. However, research indicates that this particular measure would probably be regressive, costing the poor relatively more than the rich[182]. Further research into other fiscal measures should be carried out in Ireland to assess whether they can reduce obesity levels (see Recommendations in Chapter 5).

Physical activity interventions

Physical activity interventions have multiple levels of influence on behaviour and are found to be most effective when they focus on changes in four areas: intrapersonal, social, environmental and policy[183].

Research suggests that the effectiveness of physical activity intervention programmes may be increased by the participants feeling confident about their ability to continue with the physical activities, that they enjoy the activities, that they receive encouragement and assistance from other people in their lives and that they live in areas where there is a supportive environment with convenient, attractive and safe places for physical activity[184]. Easy access to recreational facilities and programmes as well as the aesthetic qualities of neighbourhoods (such as enjoyable scenery) were related to increased physical activity[185].

School physical education programmes and community recreation programmes represent effective ways of influencing adolescent physical activity levels. In one United States study, physical activity was closely associated with environmental factors while physical inactivity was more closely related to socio-demographic factors[186]. This study found that different determinants are associated with physical activity than those associated with physical inactivity and the findings stress the importance of national level policies that are inclusive of all segments of the population.

The presence of convenient physical activity facilities has been associated with increased exercise in adults[187]. Pre-school children were more physically active where there were places nearby such as parks where they could play[188]. Research has shown that pre-school children's activity levels vary depending on the facilities and services they attend. Therefore preschool policies and practices have an important influence on the overall activity levels of the children who attend these facilities[91]. The benefits of environmental intervention policies in support of increasing physical activity are still unclear and there is a lack of comprehensive evidence on the effectiveness of these policies. Their implementation needs ongoing evaluation to measure its effect on physical activity[189].

Community intervention

While recognising the desirability of evidence-based policy, there have been relatively few adequately resourced evaluations of many potentially useful public health strategies to tackle obesity [32,190,191]. The best available evidence must therefore be sought out and used to inform policy decisions and to develop prevention and treatment strategies. A comprehensive obesity prevention programme has been introduced very recently for example in Singapore, but insufficient time has elapsed for any evaluation of long-term success to be possible. It is important for the future to build-in a properly designed action research framework for long-term assessment of policy impact, particularly for vulnerable sub-groups.

Facilitating action to address childhood obesity is complex. Screening for obesity potential may help target resources where they are most needed, but such screening also creates stigma among the children identified if they are singled out for special attention[32]. There is strong prejudice against overweight people [104, 111,] which many children are clearly aware of[112] including those as young as four years of age[113]. Care must be taken so that obesity prevention programs do not induce unhealthy slimming practices, which may lead to the development of clinical eating disorders[192], or risky behaviour such as smoking to control weight[71]. Secondly, adequate nutrition is essential for the preservation of normal growth and development. Energy restriction in obese children who were on well-controlled and supervised weight-reduction diets has led to reductions in height velocity[193]. Nonetheless, it has been shown[194] that individualised treatment with frequent monitoring can be effective without compromising growth.

The current situation requires a population health approach for adults and children in addition to the one-to-one weight-reduction management required for those who are severely overweight or with complications. This includes addressing the obesogenic environment where people live. In common with other developed countries, changing personal health practices regarding healthy eating and active living necessitates protecting people from the widespread availability of unhealthy food and beverage options in addition to sedentary activities that take up all their leisure time. However, creating environmental changes that support long-term changes in individual eating and activity habits are necessary for both adults and children if the current trends in obesity prevalence are to be tackled successfully.

Obesity prevention has been incorporated into other community-wide strategies such as the Community Prevention of Obesity in Canada[195] and the North Karelia Project, a community-based project for prevention of cardiovascular disease launched in Finland in 1972[196]. The North Karelia intervention used multiple strategies including innovative media campaigns, policy changes and environmental changes in collaboration with the food industry and agriculture. It demonstrated that a well-planned and determined community-based programme can have an effect on lifestyle and risk factors. A recent report focuses on aspects of population health that need more attention, including more upstream investment in intervention strategies[197]. This relates to ensuring a balance in intervention strategies along the continuum that stretches from individualised healthcare (downstream investments) to the introduction of policy and legislation that affects whole populations on a macro level (upstream investments). Currently, considerable effort is expended in downstream activities compared to upstream interventions[198]. **In relation to tackling the obesity problem there is growing consensus that more upstream investment is required to tackle the obesogenic environment**[199, 200, 201, 202].

Four systematic reviews have investigated the prevention of obesity and overweight in children[190, 203, 204, 205]. **There is evidence to support the use of multi-faceted school-based interventions to reduce obesity and overweight in schoolchildren, particularly girls.** These interventions included: nutrition education, physical activity promotion, reduction in sedentary behaviour, behavioural therapy, teacher training, curricular material, and modification of school meals and tuck shops[206] (see appendix D).

Three reviews have investigated the prevention of obesity in adults[203,191, 204]. The NHS CRD (1997) and Douketis et al (1999) have included the same three community-based studies in their analysis[191, 203]. The evidence from these reviews was found to be mixed and inconclusive in terms of effectiveness. Mulvihill et al (2003) found that there was inconclusive evidence regarding the effectiveness of community-based interventions (for example seminars, mailed educational packages and mass media participation) for the prevention of obesity and overweight in adults[206].

The Taskforce on Community Preventive Services in the United States supported by the Centres for Disease Control and Prevention (CDC) in that country conducted systematic reviews of community interventions to increase physical activity. Based on available evidence, the Taskforce recommended several interventions related to information dissemination and education to provide behavioural and social support for physical activity[84]. Effective interventions should include high-visibility campaigns, behaviour-change programmes, school-based education, and improved social support networks or so called 'buddy programs' to encourage physical activity. The Health Development Agency (UK) has also reviewed the effectiveness of public health interventions for increasing physical activity among adults[207] (See appendix E).

Studies have suggested that reducing television viewing, as part of a more comprehensive obesity prevention programme, may help to reduce the risk for obesity[208]. Community programmes which encourage children to play outdoors or take part in local sports or activities can remind parents and children that life is possible with little or no television. **Research has shown that parents who participate in activities with their children, organise activities and transport children to places where they can be active are the most effective supporters of their children participating in physical activity[209].**

The Review of the National Health Promotion Strategy 2004 (Department of Health and Children and NUI Galway, 2005) undertook to collect programme reports and evaluations of Regional Health Promotion Department initiatives in key topic areas such as Eating Well and Being More Active. Activities in critical areas such as sensible drinking, healthy eating and the promotion of physical activity have been substantially enhanced through national campaigns and the parallel implementation of programmes in key settings at regional level. All of these activities have served to increase the extent and reach of health promotion activities. Many of the initiatives at regional level have been subject to systematic evaluations and the findings should usefully inform the strategic development and consolidation of work in these areas. This review has highlighted that there are many excellent examples of programmes being implemented across the country, which are not being fully documented and evaluated.

Considering the potential scale of the 'obesity epidemic' and the considerable health risks associated with it, and indeed the associated economic and social consequences, the development of effective strategies to prevent obesity is a priority. **Interventions at the family and school level will need to be matched by changes in the social, environmental and cultural context so that the benefits can be sustained and enhanced.**

Management of the overweight and obese person

It is critically important that the multi-sectoral approach to obesity prevention and management in Ireland is empathetic, responsible and empowering for the significant numbers of Irish people affected.

The widespread prejudice against overweight people[104, 111] carries serious implications for psycho-social health due to the considerable social stigma associated with obesity. This can lead to isolation and humiliation of people who are overweight. It is critically important that obesity prevention and treatment initiatives tackle such prejudice and stigma so that people who are most affected by the obesity epidemic can be empowered to take action. The problem of rising obesity prevalence is not due to a lack of responsiveness by the individuals in the population. On the contrary in the United States, where the evidence of increasing obesity rates is very reliable, there is also evidence that the majority of the population are actively trying to control their weight[210]. It is important that people who are overweight or obese are encouraged to try to lose weight even when the goal of ideal weight remains elusive. **There are significant health benefits to be gained from very modest weight loss (10%) in people who remain overweight and obese[211].** Furthermore, evidence is accumulating about the beneficial effects of healthy eating and active living among people who remain overweight[212].

The management of obesity is based on evidence which demonstrates that a combination of physical, dietary and behavioural changes can improve the weight of an individual. Mulvihill and Quigley (2003) carried out an analysis of the reviews of evidence for the management of overweight and obesity[206] (see Appendix D).

There is evidence that a whole family approach is effective in managing obesity in children. Programmes which focus on the parent as being key in the behaviour change of the child were the most successful, multi-faceted family-based behaviour modification programmes which comprised diet, exercise, reducing sedentary behaviour and lifestyle counselling, with training in child management, parenting and communication skills. Laboratory-based exercise programmes were also shown to be effective in the management of childhood obesity. These programmes consisted of walking, jogging, cycle ergometry, high-repetition resistance exercise and combinations within a laboratory setting, as opposed to free-living lifestyle activity interventions. The UK Health Development Agency Review showed that there is limited evidence that behaviour modification programmes with no parental involvement are effective in the treatment of childhood obesity and overweight [206].

In adults there is evidence to support the effectiveness of low calorie diets (1,000-1,500 kcal/day), low fat (where 30% or less of total daily energy is derived from fat) combined with energy restriction, and low-fat diets alone [206]. While increased physical activity is effective in producing a moderate total weight loss, diet alone is more effective than physical activity alone. Physical activity alone, diet alone, and physical activity and diet combined are effective interventions for managing obesity in adults. Mulvihill and Quigley (2003) also found that a combination of behavioural therapy techniques in conjunction with other weight-loss approaches is effective for the treatment of adult obesity over a one-year period [206].

Weight regain, after loss, experienced by many individuals following a clinical management programme suggests that while this approach is necessary it is not sufficient on its own to reverse the incidence of obesity[202]. A population approach, on the other hand, could potentially attenuate and eventually reverse this public health problem, although this has not yet been demonstrated. This is not to suggest that only policy investments are worthy. As others have indicated[213] individual-based activities need to be balanced by broader ecological approaches to obesity prevention.

Although empirical evidence surrounding public health nutrition and physical activity interventions is limited, the issue of obesity is largely influenced by societal changes affecting eating patterns and physical activity behaviour. Under such circumstances recommendations must be drawn up using the precautionary principle since it is unethical to allow the potential harm to continue. Full proof of efficacy is not essential when considering actions to protect vulnerable groups against harm. **Policies must be introduced at a national level which support individuals in their efforts to lose weight or prevent weight gain by addressing the underlying societal factors that act as barriers to change.**

5 The way FORWARD

5 The way FORWARD

THE POLICY CHALLENGE

This report has demonstrated in preceding chapters that the determinants of diet and physical activity are complex, multi-sectoral and multi-faceted. A balance of food intake and physical activity is necessary for a healthy weight. The foods we individually consume and our participation in physical activity are the result of a complex supply and production system influenced by public policy, market forces and personal preferences, in turn dictated by our cultural traditions, beliefs and attitudes. The escalating problem of overweight and obesity is, we have shown, a global phenomenon, affecting rich and poor countries across the world. The rapidity of the rising trends, particularly in the youngest section of society, is confirmed from various sources of surveillance and lifestyle data in Ireland also. **Such evidence implies that factors outside the individual's immediate, conscious discretion are at play here.** We have also shown that there are major socio-economic trends, in the prevalence of overweight and obesity, in consumption patterns of particular food types more likely to predispose to obesity and in patterns of inactivity. An analysis of retail marketing and supply patterns implicates particular factors, such as portion size in inverse proportion to cost and containing high energy density content, as being important. We have also noted with some emphasis that modern patterns of eating out and accessing pre-prepared meals can be problematic.

All of this is further compounded by environments which are not conducive to physical activity. Poor facilities, insufficient amenities, a reduction in physical labour, increased mechanisation and personal issues surrounding self-efficacy and self-esteem are evidential factors which contribute to this complex issue. It is clear that physical activity is vital for continued good health and the prevention of many clinical conditions. From current evidence it is known that a large proportion of children and adolescents do not meet the physical activity recommendations, and despite the relationship between physical education and long-term physical activity, we do not have mandatory physical education classes. The promotion of physical activity at a national level would help to ameliorate sedentary behaviours and increase physical activity. For this to be effective environmental policies need to facilitate daily physical activity as the easy and preferred option. It is evident that all government departments, agencies and local authorities should develop proactive policies to increase the levels of physical activity and physical fitness.

The implications for a long-term effective strategy are therefore inescapable. **A population shift must be facilitated, to enable individuals to have more discretion and control in what and how much they eat, at an accessible price and with adequate opportunity to achieve energy balance by as much integrated activity in their daily routine as possible. This shift will require a change in attitude and practice, by members of the general public, by those who produce, retail and supply the market commodities in question, by healthcare providers as advocates as well as care givers, by policy makers with the power and influence to effect change, underpinned as necessary by legislation. Nothing short of this will achieve the desired benefit for most people and nothing less is acceptable in a caring, responsive society.**

A framework is required for such initiative that has at its core the rights and benefits to the individual. Health promotion is fundamentally about empowerment, whether at the individual, the community or the policy level. It cannot be ignored also that a proportion of our population, those who are currently either overweight or obese, require comprehensive clinical management programmes which promote life skills to facilitate change as part of our existing health service.

Facilitating healthy choices

People of course have a fundamental right to choose to eat what they want and to be as active as they wish. That is not the issue. The central tenet of this report is that many forces are actively impeding change for those well aware of the potential health and well-being consequences to themselves of overweight and obesity. The social change strategy is to give people meaningful choice. Our recommendations are therefore couched in these principles. The factors influencing individual choice and capacity for change occur at the level of the individual's skills and preferences, in the amenities available in the individual's immediate social environment or in settings such as the school, the workplace, and the local community services. Participation and dialogue are necessary for meaningful shifts in opinion and practice, because a top-down imposed strategy cannot be sustained for long. In the specific instance of those already tending to be overweight or with a more established weight problem the health care sector must become more proactive and vigilant in early intervention and support. Finally, if all these conditions are right, a form of 'health proofing' of public policy across a spectrum of public bodies and services will be required to put real wheels under this vehicle for change.

The Ottawa Charter for Health Promotion published in 1986 sets out these tenets of healthy public policy – supportive environments, personal skills development, re-oriented services and community participation – as fundamental for health promotion and its precepts have been adopted in many previous policy documents across a wide variety of issues[10]. The Jakarta Declaration (1997) in turn emphasised the critical role played by inter-sectoral partnership and collaboration in achieving change[11]. The agenda of the National Taskforce on Obesity is to set in motion immediate, appropriately targeted practical action and we have set out our recommendations accordingly.

Joined-up thinking

We have set out first some high-level guiding principles that we hope the Minister for Health and Children will consider in making this case to Cabinet colleagues. Ireland led the world in tackling the public health problem posed by smoking in 2004. **Our economic analysis in this report demonstrates similarly that the problem of obesity is very costly to society in human and financial terms and must be taken seriously as a resource issue.** It will be necessary to have high-level cabinet support to implement our recommendations. The approach must be proactive and inter-sectoral, which, translated into plain language, means real engagement on this issue at a practical level by the public and private sectors, as well as non-government organisations with a role to play. The motivation is to improve well-being and support people in making their choices. Joined-up thinking is a must in this situation if we are to avoid duplication of effort, cross-purpose approaches and general confusion about responsibilities. As far as possible existing strategies and agencies need to be harnessed as means of delivery on what is required. As with many lifestyle issues matters of equity and access have a powerful role to play. The least well off have the most difficulty in eating well and access to healthcare and intervention services may well pose real barriers for some in our society.

Within the public sector the range of government departments with roles to play is very considerable. It includes the Department of Health and Children itself; Agriculture and Food; Finance; Arts, Sport and Tourism; Education and Science; Environment, Heritage and Local Government; Enterprise, Trade and Employment; Social and Family Affairs; Transport; Justice,

Equality and Law Reform. We gave specific consideration to the roles such departments can play in considering our final recommendations. In many cases we felt that the implementation of what we suggest is best left to those with experience in their own sector, but in many cases also we were more explicit, in highlighting initiatives we felt were appropriate. We note also that in several of the submissions we received there was evidence already of the kind of the creative thinking necessary and we have adopted their suggestions.

Departmental roles

The following are some examples of what could be done. The Department of Finance can ensure a fundamental review of economic policy, ensure that departmental budget allocations are proofed for their likely influence on nutrition and physical activity, and commission a wider risk benefit assessment of present taxation provision. VAT could be re-examined in relation to health impact. A key Department is that of Education and Science, in facilitating within educational establishments at all levels the ethos, structure and curricula that promote physical activity and balanced eating. A core contribution of the education sector is to produce an equitable and effective general education since social inequality features so profoundly in the determinants of overweight and obesity. The Department of Arts, Sport and Tourism can facilitate a shift in how we think about activity and exercise in order to widen participation across the age and social spectrum. The Department of Agriculture and Food can ensure that best price is linked to quality and health properties of food, can support local co-operative initiatives and facilitate affordable pricing. The Department of Enterprise, Trade and Employment can revisit entitlement schemes on food production and, through its role in relation to the workplace, facilitate change in that sector too. The Department of the Environment, Heritage and Local Government can ensure a more proactive approach to planning policy, to adequate walkways and amenities, can ensure public transport provision is explicit in that planning process. The Department of Social and Family Affairs is influential in relation to many social services, ranging from school meals, to local funding of community schemes and welfare payments that could be reviewed for realistic affordability to low-income families of healthy option foods. The departments of the Environment and of Transport each have a profound influence on the quality and conducive nature of the physical environment in which we live.

The Department of Health and Children through the newly reformed health services structure has a flagship role to play in re-oriented service delivery. It is important that healthy lifestyles are supported and encouraged throughout life, beginning from the earliest years. All contacts with the health services, both scheduled and opportunistic should be used as opportunities to promote and encourage healthy eating and active living. There are in place public health systems which monitor and support children and families in the three years after discharge from maternity services and through the primary schools system with the immunisation schemes. These are opportunities to access children and their families and they should be used as such to support and promote healthy eating and active living. Although prevention is key in these years early detection of overweight and obesity is important so that the children and adolescents can be supported in making healthy choices. The school/education setting is important because the majority of children are in school for at least their first two decades and so they can be accessed for health education and promotion.

Monitoring and surveillance are essential tools in the implementation of national strategies for healthy diets and physical activity (WHO, 2004)[12]. There is a need for long term and continuous monitoring of the risk factors, including overweight and obesity, because such data can provide the basis of analysis of changes in prevalence which could be attributable to changes in policies and strategies. Trends in overweight and obesity, especially in children, should be closely monitored because of their public health importance and because it is important that programmes and policies implemented to address overweight and obesity are evaluated for their effectiveness. Surveillance can be based on repeated surveys or, for children, on data from child health or growth monitoring programmes. Identification of populations and geographical areas at risk of overweight and obesity may help formulate policy and promote local programmes designed to improve the health of the community (WHO, 2004)[12].

The Framework set out below serves as a model for action, through which we organise our recommendations.

Figure 5.1: Framework for obesity prevention[214]

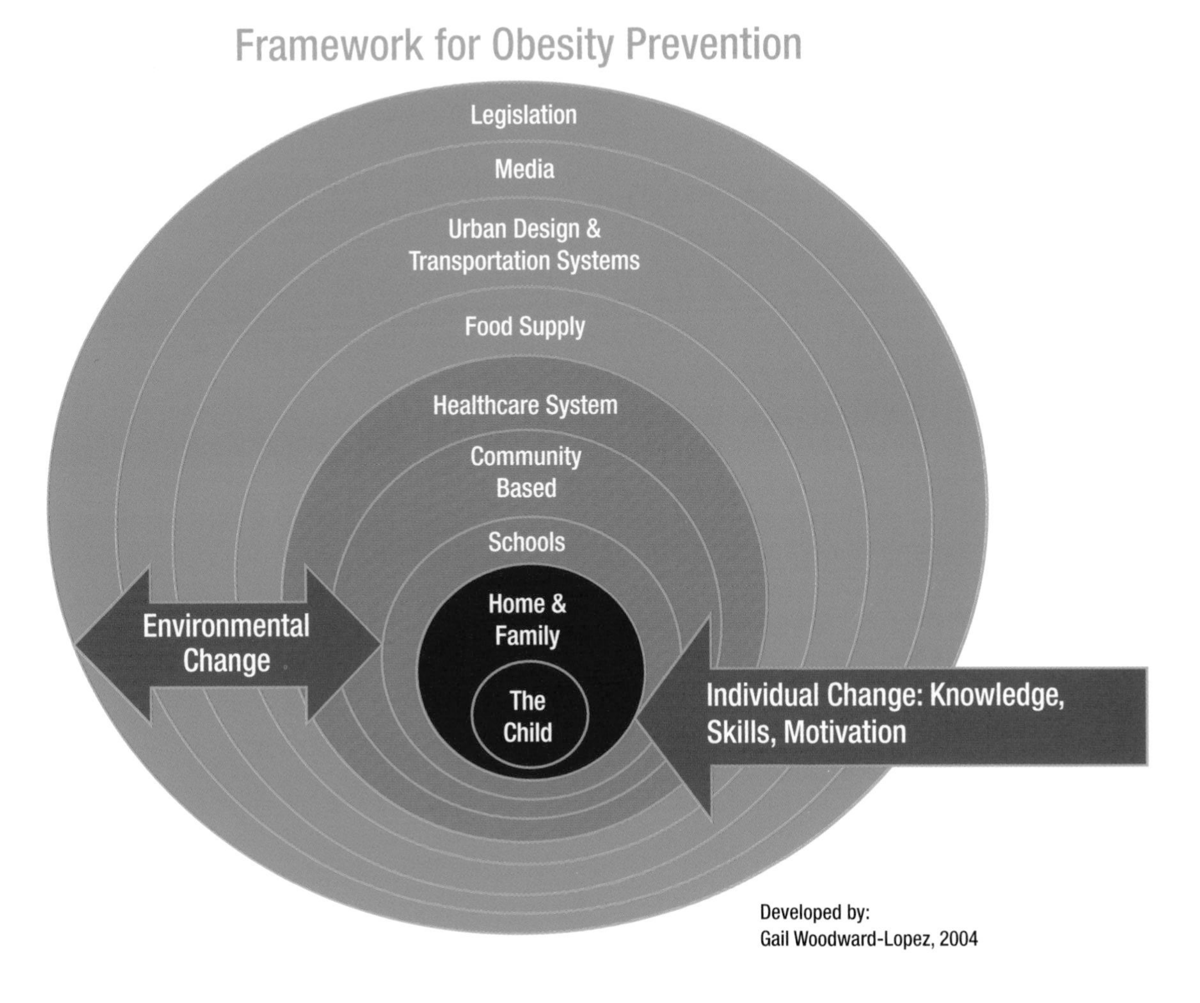

VISION

An Irish society that enables people through health promotion, prevention and care to achieve and maintain healthy eating and active living throughout their lifespan

High-level goals (overriding principles)

- The Taoiseach's Office will ensure that an integrated, consistent and proactive approach will be taken across all government departments, agencies and public bodies in addressing the problem of overweight/obesity.
- The private sector has an important role; it acknowledges it has a responsibility and will be proactive in addressing the issue of overweight/obesity.
- The public sector, the private sector and the community and voluntary sectors should work in partnership to promote healthy eating and active living to address overweight/obesity.
- Individuals should be personally empowered to tackle overweight and obesity and sensitive interventions should be developed to support them.

The National Taskforce on Obesity has used the following **principles** as a framework to its recommendations:

- Formulating, implementing and monitoring of **healthy public policy** and the promotion of **social responsibility** for overweight and obesity.
- Encouraging **supportive environmental measures** and securing an **infrastructure** which improves health.
- Strengthening **community action** and increasing **community capacity.**
- Developing **personal skills** and **empowering** the individual.
- **Reorientating** the public services, including the health services, to advocate for health.
- Increasing **investments for health** development.
- Expanding **partnerships** for health.

NATIONAL TASKFORCE ON OBESITY RECOMMENDATIONS

1 High-level government

1 The Taoiseach's office should take the lead responsibility and provide an integrated and consistent proactive approach to addressing overweight and obesity and to the implementation, monitoring and evaluation of the National Strategy on Obesity in conjunction with all government departments, relevant bodies and agencies, industry and consumer groups.

2 All state agencies and government departments, as part of a health impact assessment, need to develop, prioritise and evaluate schemes and policies (including public procurement) that encourage healthy eating and active living, especially those aimed at children and vulnerable groups.

3 The Department of Finance should carry out research to examine the influence of fiscal policies on consumer purchasing and their impact on overweight and obesity, for example risk-benefits assessment of taxation that supports healthy eating and active living, subsidies for healthy food such as fruit and vegetables.

4 Ireland should play an advocacy role within the European Union to reform policies relating to healthy eating and active living among those that govern activities relating to global trade and the regulation of marketing and advertising of food to children.

5 The Taoiseach's office, as part of the proactive approach in addressing overweight and obesity, should seek the views of children and young people and those members of the population who are, at present, overweight/obese.

2 Education sector

1 All schools, as part of their school development planning, should be encouraged to develop consistent school policies to promote healthy eating and active living, with the necessary support from the Department of Education and Science. Such policies should address opportunities for physical activity, what is being provided in school meals, including breakfast clubs, school lunches and, in the case of primary schools in partnership with parents, children's lunch boxes.

2 The emphasis in all schools should be on increased physical activity including participation in sports.

3 With a view to achieving the optimum 60 minutes of physical activity per day recommendation (excluding PE time) every child should be enabled, through restructuring the school day if necessary, to achieve a minimum of 30 minutes dedicated physical activity every day in all educational settings.

4 All schools should meet the minimum requirement of two hours of physical education per week delivered by appropriately qualified staff.

5 The Department of Education and Science should prioritise the provision and maintenance of physical education and physical activity facilities to address the issue of equity and access in all schools.

6 The Department of Education and Science should provide resources for adequate teacher training to support healthy eating and active living.

7 Nutrition and physical activity levels of school children should be seen as part of the duty of care of each school, for example in relation to catering for school meals, policy on vending machines, and provision of fresh drinking water.

8 Vending machines should be banned in primary schools and those in the food and drink industry who have already voluntarily prohibited the placing of vending machines in primary schools should be supported.

9 A clear code of practice in relation to the provision and content of vending machines in post-primary schools should be developed by industry, the Department of Education and Science and schools' representative bodies.

10 The Schools Inspectorate in the course of its evaluation of activities in schools should focus on the prevention of obesity and should further develop its indicators to do this.

11 The restructured senior cycle curriculum should incorporate Social, Personal and Health Education, and focus on the life skills and empowerment necessary for the prevention of obesity.

12 Home-school-community coordinators should incorporate 'healthy life skills' within the wider framework of home visitation and should promote courses and classes for parents, where appropriate.

13 All post-primary schools should be encouraged to engage with their student councils and parents' associations in promoting the concept of 'healthy eating and active living'.

14 All third-level colleges and institutions should be encouraged to adopt the 'health promoting college' concept and to actively address issues concerning healthy eating, drinking behaviour and sedentary lifestyle patterns.

15 The national parents' organisations for primary and post-primary schools should work with parents and support them in encouraging healthy eating and active living.

16 A national, regularly reviewed code of practice must be developed in relation to industry sponsorship and funding of activities in schools and local communities.

17 Evidence-based intervention programmes should be introduced to all primary schools on a consistent basis in line with exemplars of good practice such as NEAPS[215] and the Food Dude programme[216].

18 Curricula in catering training colleges must put greater emphasis on healthy food options.

19 Every child should receive a safe and active passage to school through the provision of safe walkways, cycleways or transport.

20 Schools should develop increasing opportunities for physical activity that are inclusive and that are appropriate to age, gender, and ability, such as those that concentrate on increasing physical activity among teenage girls.

21 Skills programmes which teach and develop training in basic food preparation and budgeting should be introduced in schools.

22 The health/immunisation programme in national schools should be used as an opportunity to work in partnership with parents and children in developing life skills which support healthy eating and active living. This programme should also be used as an opportunity to detect, by measurement, children who are at risk of overweight and underweight.

3 Social and community sectors

1 The Department of Social and Family Affairs should review social welfare (assistance) payments to take account of the relatively high cost of healthy foods for socially disadvantaged groups.

2 Access to a healthy diet (for example fruit and vegetables) should be included as an indicator to measure food poverty as part of the National Anti-Poverty Strategy/Inclusion process.

3 The Health Service Executive in the implementation of the Child Care (Pre-School Services) Regulations 1996 and (Amendment) Regulations1997 should ensure that pre-school services support healthy eating and active living.

4 The Department of Justice, Equality and Law Reform should ensure that grant recipients under the Equal Opportunities Childcare Programme provide confirmation that they are in compliance with the statutory requirements in relation to healthy eating and active living.

5 The Department of Arts, Sport and Tourism should co-ordinate with the Department of Education and Science the shared use of sports and physical activity facilities between schools and communities.

6 The Department of Arts, Sport and Tourism should focus on increasing physical activity for all members of the community and respond appropriately to developing trends.

7 The Department of Community, Rural and Gaeltacht Affairs should facilitate strengthening the capacity of communities to address health related issues at a national and local level.

8 Peer-led community development programmes should be fostered and developed to encourage healthy eating and active living. These programmes should be prioritised for lower socio-economic groups, ethnic minority groups, early school leavers, people with learning and physical disabilities and they should be based on the principle of developing self-esteem and empowerment such as is evident for example in the community mothers programme[217].

9 Community skills-based programmes should be developed which provide skills such as food preparation, household budgeting, and those skills which have the potential to promote physical activity.

10 Building on the work undertaken by community groups, community initiatives should be developed to tackle the issues of food poverty and accessibility through local food programmes and co-operatives.

11 Parents should be encouraged and supported by relevant agencies to partake in physical activities with their children.

12 Existing and future parenting courses within communities should develop and implement healthy eating and active living education as part of their programmes.

13 Groups representing older people should support and encourage national programmes for healthy eating and for physical and sporting activities among their members.

4 Health sector

1 The health services, in their strategic planning and delivery, should advocate and lead a change in emphasis from the primacy of individual responsibility to environments that support healthy food choices and regular physical activity.

2 Supporting the population in healthy eating and active living, in the prevention of overweight and obesity, should be a key goal of health services and healthcare providers.

3 The health services should recognise maintenance of a healthy weight as an important health issue, and measurement of height, weight, waist circumference and calculation of BMI should be part of routine clinical healthcare practice in primary care and in hospitals.

4 An individual's interaction with healthcare services should be an opportunity to develop life skills and foster self-efficacy in support of healthy eating, active living and positive self-image.

5 A national database of growth measurements (height, weight, waist circumference, BMI) for children and adults should be developed by the Population Health Directorate in order to monitor prevalence trends of growth, overweight and obesity. The database can be created by developing the surveillance systems that are already established and by expanding these systems to collect the required data, for example the national health and lifestyle surveys, established longitudinal research projects and the school health surveillance system.

6 Individuals who have a BMI over 25kg/m^2 and who choose to manage their weight, can do so in partnership with their healthcare provider, using the Treatment Algorithim (page 9, Supplement). Individuals with a BMI in the normal range should be enabled to monitor their progress with follow-up measurements every three years.

7 An education and training programme for health professionals in the appropriate and sensitive management of overweight and obesity should be developed and implemented. Programmes should include training in developing life skills for healthy eating and active living, counselling, readiness to change/brief intervention, and standardised measuring techniques. Primary care teams should be the focus of the initial education and training drive.

8 A practical framework for implementation of the education and training programme which would address the constraints of current primary care workload and practices should be developed. Incentives such as additional study leave, bonus Continuing Medical Education accreditation and payment may have to be considered.

9 Detection, prevention and treatment programs should be evaluated to ensure that they are being implemented as planned and that they are effective. This evaluation must include stakeholder input at all stages to ensure that programmes are being tailored to meet the needs of the target population.

10 The curriculum for undergraduates and postgraduates in relevant health sciences should provide training in appropriate and sensitive obesity prevention and management.

11 Individuals at risk of developing an eating disorder should be assessed proactively with the aid of a simple screening tool developed by relevant support groups and appropriate experts.

12 A North/South communication and public awareness programme on overweight and obesity should be developed in conjuction with and regularly evaluated by the HSE in partnership with the Northern Ireland Department of Health, appropriate food agencies, government representatives, non-governmental agencies, consumers and appropriate industries. Consistent, clear media messages should be sensitive and appropriate to culture, age and gender.

13 The guidelines for physical activity, and for food and nutrition required for good health should be reviewed by the Population Health Directorate, in partnership with the appropriate food agencies, consumer and community groups, relevant government bodies, NGOs, and industry, to include the prevention and management of overweight and obesity.

14 All guidelines for physical activity, food and nutrition should be developed according to age and gender and should be independently proofed by the relevant authorities to ensure that they are appropriate.

15 To ensure best practice, consistency and the safety of the population, all overweight and obesity prevention and management strategies should be co-ordinated and regularly reviewed by the Population Health Directorate of the HSE.

16 Individuals should be facilitated in choosing to manage their health and weight effectively by identifying their needs and possible risks. This should be achieved through partnership with their healthcare provider.

17 Antenatal visits are an opportunity to empower parents and their families to develop life skills which support healthy eating and active living. They should encompass family goals, such as healthy weights, which are regularly discussed.

18 The choice of a mother to breastfeed and the skills required to breastfeed exclusively for the recommended six months should be supported ante-natally and postpartum.

19 The postpartum check presents a further opportunity for the public health nurse, parents and their families to discuss and facilitate health choices. To support the family in maintaining healthy weights, key measurements, such as child's weight/length and the mother's BMI, should be recorded to enable self-management.

20 The primary care vaccination visits and public health nurse visits carried out during the first three years of a child's life is another opportunity to engage with families, working in partnership with parents to assess and monitor changes in the BMI of the parents and the height/length of children and to identify skills to overcome barriers to change.

21 All children and parents have the opportunity through the school health services to develop self-capacity in relation to healthy eating and active living and this should include the opportunity to have a growth assessment for overweight or underweight. Assessments should be carried out on school entry (4-5 years) and then at regular intervals (for example 9-11 years and 14-16 years) throughout the child's development. Children and their families should be enabled to make appropriate changes by working in partnership with the relevant professionals, in particular the primary care team and dietary and physical activity professionals.

22 Individuals' capacities in choosing to manage their health and well-being are strengthened with the knowledge of their height, weight, waist circumference and BMI. This can be achieved in partnership with their GP and health care providers in the primary care team.

23 Individuals should be facilitated in the management of their health, in the community setting, by the provision of opportunistic standardised height/weight measurement in leisure centres, sports clubs and recreational facilities. This should be developed in partnership with the relevant health services.

24 Formative research should be carried out to ensure programs are being implemented as planned. This must include stakeholder input at developmental, implementation and evaluation stages to ensure programs are being tailored to meet the needs of target population.

5 Food, commodities, production and supply

1 The Department of Enterprise, Trade and Employment, the Department of Health and Children, together with the private sector and consumer groups should immediately take multi-sectoral action on the marketing and advertising of products that contribute to weight gain, in particular those aimed at children.

2 The Department of Agriculture and Food should review policies in partnership with other government departments to promote access to healthy food. Such policies should encompass positive discrimination in the provision of grants and funding to local industry in favour of healthy products.

3 The Department of Agriculture and Food together with the Department of Health and Children should promote the implementation of evidence-based healthy eating interventions.

4 Guidelines for food and nutrition labelling should be reviewed and further developed by the appropriate food agencies in conjunction with industry and consumer groups, to ensure that labelling is accurate, consistent, user-friendly and contains information on portion sizes and nutrient content.

5 There should be a rigorous and regular review of all products that claim to support weight-loss. Food and beverage slimming products should be reviewed by the appropriate food agencies, while medical products should be reviewed by the Irish Medicines Board.

6 A single representative industry body should be established to implement and monitor consistently the relevant Taskforce recommendations as they relate to that sector and to specifically collaborate on issues relating to partnership in this strategy.

7 The food and drinks manufacturing industry, the retail sector, the catering industry and the suppliers to these should promote research and development investment in healthier food choices.

8 The food and drinks industry should be consistent in following the lead of those who have already abandoned extra-large-value individual portion sizes.

9 A practical healthy nutrition programme should be established by the health services, the appropriate food agencies and the catering institutions to ensure that all catering facilities provide healthy options.

6 Physical environment

1. The Department of the Environment, Heritage and Local Government should develop coherent planning policies for urban/rural housing, transport, amenity spaces and workplace settings to encourage spontaneous increases in physical activity in adults and children.

2. The Department of Enterprise, Trade and Employment should ensure that future safety, health and welfare at work legislation promotes and protects health with a particular emphasis on healthy eating and active living.

3. The Irish Financial Services Regulatory Authority should examine the high costs of public liability and their impact on physical activity. It should foster initiatives to address these costs.

4. The Department of Enterprise, Trade and Employment, the electronic leisure industry and consumer groups should review the design, production and marketing policies surrounding products that impact on healthy eating and active living, particularly in relation to children.

5. The Department of Transport and the Department of the Environment should apply a specifically designated percentage of all road budgets to the construction of safe walkways and cycleways.

6. The Department of Transport should increase the provision of safe and efficient public transport and set targets for the reduction of car use.

7. Local authorities should ensure that their mission statements, corporate plans and planning policies take account of their impact on healthy living.

8. Local authorities should work in partnership with community groups to actively promote sporting and leisure opportunities that support active living.

9. Local authorities, bearing in mind regional variations and the demography of their populations, should ensure that sports, recreational, leisure, and play facilities are available, accessible and equitable to all members of the public.

10. Local authorities should prioritise pedestrianisation and cycling and ensure that there is adequate provision for these amenities.

11. Local authorities in partnership with local communities and the gardaí should ensure the provision and maintenance of safe and accessible green spaces for physical activity. They should be supported by government in this and related work.

12. The Department of Arts, Sport, and Tourism should ensure that sports, leisure and social organisations receiving funding are encouraged to have regard to the health of their members, for example in terms of catering, sponsorship etc. Funding should be proofed, evaluated and monitored by nationally recognised sports and physical activity groups.

13 Local authorities should ensure that their leisure and activity centres develop policies that promote healthy eating.

14 Private sector organisations that promote physical activity, such as leisure centres and gyms, should develop policies that reflect healthy eating.

15 The private leisure industry should be encouraged to make its facilities more accessible to lower socio-economic and minority groups through partnership with local communities, local authorities and health boards.

16 Workplaces in both the private and public sectors should provide an environment that empowers individuals to make healthy food choices and presents opportunities during work hours to partake in physical activity, opportunities such as flexible working hours, reduced rates for gym membership, incentives for cycling or walking to work, access to shower and changing facilities.

17 Occupational health and wellness services, should include the option of weight status screening of employees and encourage staff to participate in work-based healthy eating and active living programs.

18 All employers should make arrangements to facilitate mothers who choose to breastfeed on their return to the workplace.

19 Every workplace should have a healthy work-life balance policy which is regularly reviewed. These policies should form part of the national partnership agreements. The social partners must place a greater emphasis on health promotion as part of the national work-life balance policy. All policies and regulations currently in existence in this area must be fully implemented.

20 Community development programmes which encourage healthy eating and active living should be developed in partnership with local authorities and businesses. These programmes should be prioritised for lower socio-economic groups, ethnic minority groups, early school leavers, and people with learning and physical disabilities.

References

1.Department of Health And Children." Building Healthier Hearts" :Report of the Cardiovascular Health Strategy Group. DOHC 1999.

2.Department of Health & Children (2000) The National Health Promotion Strategy 2000-2005. The stationery office. Dublin.

3. Department of Health and Children (1991) Nutrition Health Promotion: Framework for Action. The stationary office, Dublin

4. Nutrition Advisory Group, Recommendations for a Food and Nutrition Policy for Ireland, The stationary office, Dublin , 1995.

5. Hamilton, N. & Bhatti, T. (1996). Population Health Promotion: An integrated model of population health and health promotion. Ottawa, Health Canada: Health Promotion Development Division.

6. Community Prevention of Obesity Steering Committee (2003). Community Prevention of Obesity: Framework for Action. Calgary, Calgary Health Region.

7. Department of Health and Children (2001) Quality and Fairness: A Health System for you. National Health Strategy. The stationary office, Dublin.

8. National Children's Office (2004) Ready, Steady, Play : A national play policy.The stationery office, Dublin.

9. Department of Health and Children (1994) A National Breastfeeding Policy for Ireland. The stationery office, Dublin.

10. World Health Organisation. (1996) Ottawa Charter for Health Promotion, WHO, Geneva.

11. World Health Organisation. (1997).The Jakarta Declaration on Leading Health Promotion into the 21st Century, WHO, Geneva

12 World Health Organisation (2004) Global Strategy on Diet, physical activity and health.

13. Conway, B. & Rene, A. (2004) Obesity as a disease: No lightweight matter. Obesity Reviews; 5: 145-151.

14. World Health Organisation. (1998).Obesity – preventing and managing the global epidemic. Report of a WHO consultation on Obesity. WHO, Geneva.

15. National Institutes of Health (NIH), National Heart, Lung and Blood Institute (NHLBI). Clinical guidelines on the identification, evaluation, and treatment of overweight and obesity in adults: Evidence Report. HHS, Public Health Services (PHS); 1998. http://www.nhlbi.nih.gov/guidelines/obesity/ob_home.htm

16. Irish Universities Nutrition Alliance (2001) North/South Ireland Food Consumption Survey. http://www.iuna.net/survey_contents.htm

17. Jeffrey, A.N., Voss, L.D., Metcalf, B.S., Alba, S. and Wilkin, T.J. (2005) Parents' awareness of overweight in themselves and their children: cross sectional study with a cohort (EarlyBird 21). British Medical Journal; 330:23-24.

18. World Health Organisation. (2003) Controlling the global obesity epidemic. http://www.who.int/nut/obs.htm

19. Rigby N (2002) The Global Challenge of Obesity and the International Obesity Taskforce. International Union of Nutritional Sciences http://www.iuns.org/features/obesity/obesity.htm

20. National Centre for Health Statistics, Centre for Disease Control and Prevention (2004) Healthy, United States, 2004. Hyattsville, Maryland.

21. International Obesity Task Force (IOTF) and European Association for the Study of Obesity (EASO) Position paper; Obesity in Europe – the case for action. London, 2002 www.iotf.org

22. Scholes S, Prescott A, Bajekal M. Health Survey for England: Health & lifestyle indicators for Strategic Health Authorities 1994-2002 Department of Health(UK), 2004.

23. Northern Ireland Statistics and Research Agency (1997) Health and Wellbeing Survey. Central Survey Unit: Northern Ireland Statistics and Research Agency.

24. Pomerleau J, Pudule I, Grinberga D, Kadziauskiene K, Abaravicius A, Bartkeviciute R, Vaask S, Robertson A, McKee M (2000) Patterns of body weight in the Baltic Republics.Public Health Nutr;3(1):3-10.

25. International Obesity Taskforce (IOTF) (2003). Position paper: Waiting for a green light for health?- Europe at the crossroads for diet and disease.
http://www.iotf.org/media/euobesity2.pdf

26. Irish Nutrition and Dietetic Institute (1990) The Irish National Nutrition Survey. Dublin: INDI.

27. Kelleher C, Nic Gabhainn S, Friel S, (1999) The National Health and Lifestyle Surveys: Survey of Lifestyle, Attitudes and Nutrition (SLÁN 1998) and The Irish Health Behaviour in School-Aged Children Survey (HBSC).Centre for Health Promotion Studies, NUI Galway.

28. Kelleher C, Nic Gabhainn S, Friel S, Corrigan H, Nolan G, Sixsmith J, Walsh O, Cooke M. (2003) The National Health and Lifestyle Surveys: Survey of Lifestyle, Attitudes and Nutrition (SLÁN 2002) and The Irish Health Behaviour in School-Aged Children Survey (HBSC).Centre for Health Promotion Studies, NUI Galway & The Department of Public Health Medicine and Epidemiology, UCD.

29. Hayes, K., Shiely, F., Murrin, C.M., Nolan, G. & Kelleher, C.C. (2004) A comparison of self-reported and clinically measured body mass index in Irish adults. Proceedings of the Nutrition Society (In Press)

30. McCarthy, S.N., Harrington, K.E., Kiely, M., Flynn, A., Robson, P.J., Livingstones, M.B.E. & Gibney, M.J. (2001) Analyses of the anthropometic data from the North/South Ireland Food Consumption Survey. Public Health Nutrition; 4(5A): 1099-1106.

31. Centres for Disease Control and Prevention (2002) CDC growth training modules: Using BMI-for-age charts
http://www.cdc.gov/nccdphp/dnpa/growthcharts/training/modules/overview.htm

32. Lobstein, T., Baur, L. & Uauy, R for International Obesity TaskForce. (2004) Obesity in children and young people: a crisis in public health. Obesity Reviews; 5 (Suppl.1): 4-85.

33. Cole TJ, Freeman JV, Preece MA (1995) Body mass index reference curves for the UK, 1990. Archives of Disease in Childhood; 73(1): 25-29.

34. Cole TJ, Bellizzi MC, Flegal KM, Dietz WH. (2000) Establishing a standard definition for child overweight and obesity worldwide: international survey. British Medical Journal; 320:1-6.

35. Popkin BM, Richards MK, Montiero CA (1996) Stunting is associated with overweight in children of four nations that are undergoing the nutrition transition. Journal of Nutrition;126(12):3009-16.

36. National Centre for Health Statistics (NCHS), Centre for Disease Control and Prevention (CDC).Prevalence of overweight among children and adolescents: United States, 1999. www.cdc.gov/nchs/products/pubs/pubd/hestats/over99fig1.htm

37. Lobstein T. and Frelut ML. (2003) Prevalence of overweight among children in Europe. Obesity Reviews 4 (4): 195-200.

38. Stamatakis, E.(2004) Health Survey for England 2002 : The Health of children and young people (Eds. Sproston & Primatesta). Stationery Office, London. http://www.official-documents.co.uk/document/deps/doh/survey02/hcyp/hcyp01.htm

39. Griffin AC, Younger KM, Flynn MA (2004) Assessment of obesity and fear of fatness among inner city Dublin school children in a one-year follow-up study. Public Health Nutrition; 7(6):729-35.

40. Whelton H., Crowley E., Kelleher V., Perry I, Cronin M (In press 2005) North South Survey of Height, Weight and Body Mass Index in Ireland, 2002. Department of Health and Children, Dublin and Department of Health, Social Services and Personal Safety, Northern Ireland.

41. Mulvihill, C., Nemeth, A. & Vereecken, C. (2004) Body image, weight control and body weight. In Young People's Health in Context. Health Behaviour in School-Aged Children (HBSC) study: international report from the 2001/2002 survey. Currie et al. (Editors). WHO, Copenhagen, 2004. (www.hbsc.org).

42. World Health Organisation. (2003) Diet, Nutrition and the prevention of chronic diseases. Report of a joint WHO/FAO expert consultation. WHO. Geneva. (WHO Technical Report Series, No. 916).

43. Rolls, B.J. (2000) The role of energy density in the overconsumption of fat. Journal of Nutrition; 130: 269S-271S.

44. Prentice, A.M. & Jebb, S.A. (2003) Fast foods, energy density and obesity: a possible mechanistic link. Obesity Reviews; 4: 187-194.

45. U.S Dept of Health and Human Services (USDHHS) and US Department of Agriculture (2005) Dietary Guidelines for Americans. U.S. Government Printing Office, Washington. http://www.healthierus.gov/dietaryguidelines/

46. McCarthy, S.N., Robson, P.J., Flynn, A. & Gibney, M.J. (2002) Health and Lifestyle variables that predict body mass index and body fat distribution in a nationally representative sample of Irish adults.Proceedings of the Nutrition Society; 61:169A.

47. National Nutrition Surveillance Centre (2003) Annual Report: Dietary Habits of the Irish Population – Results from SLÁN. Government Publications Office, Dublin.

48. Astrup A, Buemann B, Flint A, Raben A.(2002) Low-fat diets and energy balance: Cow does the evidence stand in 2002? Proceedings of the Nutrition Society;61(2):299-309. Review.

49. Astrup, A. (1999) Macronutrient balances and obesity: The role of diet and physical activity. Public Health Nutrition; 2(3a): 341-347.

50. Heitmann, B.L. & Lissner, L. (1995) Dietary underreporting by obese individuals – is it specific or non-specific? British Medical Journal; 311 (7011): 986-9.

51. Eurodiet (2000) Eurodiet Core Report Nutrition and Diet for Healthy Lifestyles in Europe: Science and Policy Implications. www.eurodiet.med.uoc.gr

52. Willet WC. (1998) Is dietary fat a major determinant of body fat? American Journal of Clinical Nutrition;67:S565–625

53. Brand-Miller JC, Holt SHA, Pawlak DB, McMillan J.(2002) Glycemic index and obesity. American Journal of Clinical Nutrition;76(suppl):281S–5S.

54. Gross, L.S., Li. L., Ford, E.S. & Liu, S. (2004) Increased consumption of refined carbohydrates and the epidemic of type 2 diabetes in the United States: an ecologic assessment. American Journal of Clinical Nutrition; 79: 774-779.

55. Howarth NC, Saltzman E, Roberts SB (2001) Dietary fibre and weight regulation. Nutrition Reviews; 59: 129-139.

56. Yeomans, M.R. (2004) Effects of alcohol on food energy intake in human subjects:evidence for passive and active over-consumption of energy. British Journal of Nutrition; 92: S31-34.

57. Swinburn, B.A., Caterson, I., Seidell, J.C. & James, W.P.T (2004) Diet, nutrition and the prevention of excess weight gain and obesity. Public Health Nutrition; 7: 123-146.

58. Strategic Task Force on Alcohol (2002) Interim Report. Department of Health And Children, Dublin.

59. Guthrie, J.F., Lin, B.H. & Frazao, E. (2002) Role of food prepared away from home in the American diet, 1977-78 versus 1994-96: Changes and consequences. Journal of Nutrition Education and Behaviour; 34(3):140-150.

60. Jeffrey RW, French SA. (1998) Epidemic obesity in the United States: are fast foods and television viewing contribution? American Journal of Public Health; 88:277-280.

61. Fort, M (2003) The death of cooking. In Food-the way we eat now. The Guardian May 10: Supplement issue 1:11.

62. Nolan, G., Murrin, C.M., Shiely, F., Corrigan, H., NicGabhainn, Friel, S. & Kelleher, C.C. (2004) Consumption patterns of junk foods in young Irish people in relation to body mass index. Proceedings of the Nutrition Society (In press).

63. Ludwig DS, Peterson KE, Gortmaker SL. (2001) Relation between consumption of sugar-sweetened drinks and childhood obesity: a prospective, observational analysis. Lancet; 357: 505-508.

64. Harnack L, Stang J, Story M (1999) Soft drink consumption among US children and adolescents: nutritional consequences. Journal of the American Dietetic Association; 99: 436-41.

65. Mattes RD (1996)Dietary compensation by humans for supplemental energy provided as ethanol or carbohydrate in fluids. Physiology and Behaviour;59(1):179-87.

66. Nielsen, S.J. & Popkin, B.M. (2003) Patterns and trends in food portion sizes, 1977-1998. Journal of the American Medical Association; 289 (4): 450-453.

67. McCarthy, S.N., Robson, P.J., Livingstone, M.B.E., Kiely, M., Flynn, A., Cran, G.W. & Gibney, M.J. Associations between the portion size of food consumed and excess adiposity in Irish adults: towards the development of food based dietary guidelines for reducing the prevalence of overweight and obesity (submitted for publication).

68. McCrory, M.A., Suen, V.M.M. & Roberts, S.B. (2002) Biobehavioural influences on energy intake and adult weight gain. Journal of Nutrition; 132:3830S-3845S.

69. Dykes J, Brunner EJ, Martikainen PT, Wardle J.(2004) Socioeconomic gradient in body size and obesity among women: the role of dietary restraint, disinhibition and hunger in the Whitehall II study. International Journal of Obesity Related Metabolic Disorders; 28(2): 262-268.

70. Broderick D & Shiel G. Diet & Activity Patterns of Children in Primary Schools in Ireland. St. Patrick's College, Dublin, 2000.

71. Klesges, R. C., K. D. Ward, et al. (1998). The prospective relationships between smoking and weight in a young biracial cohort: the coronoary artery risk development in young adults study. Journal of Consulting and Clinical Psychology 66: 987-993.

72. Ryan, Y. M., M. J. Gibney, et al. (1998). The pursuit of thinness: A Study of Dublin schoolgirls aged 15 years. International Journal of Obesity 22: 486-488.

73. Eid, E. E. (1970). Follow-up study of physical growth of children who had excessive weight gain in the first six months of life. British Medical Journal 2(74-76).

74. Stettler, N., Zemel, B. S., Kumanyika, S., Stallings, V. A. (2002). Infant weight gain and childhood overweight status in a multicenter, cohort study. Pediatrics 109(No.2): 194-199.

75. Stettler, N., Kumanyika, S., Solomon, H. K., Zemel, B. S., Stallings, V. A. (2003). Rapid weight gain during infancy and obesity in young adulthood in a cohort of African Americans. American Journal of Clinical Nutrition 77: 1374-1378.

76. Bergmann, K. E., Bergmann, R. L., von Kries, R., Bohm, O., Richter, R., Deudenhausen, J. W., Wahn, U. (2003). Early determinants of childhood overweight and adiposity in a birth cohort study: role of breastfeeding. International Journal of Obesity. 27: 162-172.

77. Gillman, M.W., Rifas-Shiman, S.L., Camargo, C.A., Berkey, C.S., Frazier, A.L., Rockett, H.R.H., Field, A.E. & Colditz, G.A. (2001) Risk of overweight among adolescents who were breastfed as infants. Journal of the American Medical Association; 285: 2461-2467.

78. Zimmet, P. & Thomas, C.R. (2003) Genotype, obesity and cardiovascular disease – has technical and social advancement outstripped evolution? Journal of Internal Medicine; 254:114-125.

79. Neel, J.V. (1962) Human population genetics, 1961. Acta Geneticae medica et Gemellologiael; 11:263-268.

80. U.S. Department of Health and Human Services (USDHHS) The Surgeon General's Call to Action to Prevent and Decrease Overweight and Obesity. United States Department of Health and Human Services, Washington. 2004

81. Caspersen CJ, Powell KE, Christenson GM (1985). Physical activity, exercise, and physical fitness: definitions and distinctions for health-related research. Public Health Rep. 1985 Mar-Apr;100(2):126-31

82. (The) President's Council on Physical Fitness and Sports (2000)Research Digest 3, 12; December.

83. Booth, F.W., Chakravarthy, M.V., Gordon, S.E. & Spangenburg, E.E. (2002) Waging war on physical inactivity: using modern molecular ammunition against an ancient enemy. Journal of Applied Physiology; 93(1):3-30.

84. Centres for Disease Control and Prevention (2001). Increasing physical activity: a report on recommendations of the Task Force on Community Preventive Services. MMWR2001;50(No. RR-18):1-16.

85. Wilk E. & Jansen J. (2004).Lifestyle-related risks: are trends in Europe converging? Journal of Royal Institute of Public Health.

86. World Health Organisation (2002). The world health report: reducing risks, promoting healthy life. WHO, Geneva.

87. Gregory J, Lowe S et al (2000) National Diet and Nutrition Survey: young people aged 4 to 18 years, HMSO: London

88. Rowe, N & Champion, R (2000) Young people and sport in England. National Survey 1999. Sport England, London.

89. Parliamentary Office of Science and Technology (2003) Childhood Obesity. Postnote, September, number 205. Parliamentary Office of Science and Technology, London. http://www.parliament.uk/post/pn205.pdf

90. U.S. Department of Health and Human Services (USDHHS). Healthy People 2010. 2nd ed. With Understanding and Improving Health and Objectives for Improving Health. 2 vols. Washington, DC: U.S. Government Printing Office, November 2000.

91. Pate, R.R., Freedson, P.S., Sallis, J.F., Taylor, W.C., Sirard, J., Trost, S.G., Dowda, M.(2002) Compliance with physical activity guidelines: prevalence in a population of children and youth. Annals of Epidemiology; 12(5): 303-308.

92. Woods, C., Foley, E., O'Gorman, D., Kearney, J. & Moyna, N. (2004) The Take PART Study: Physical Activity Research for Teenagers. A Report for the East Coast Area Health Board by Centre for Sport Science and Health, Dublin City University.

93. Boreham C. & Riddoch C. (2001) The physical activity, fitness and health of children.Journal of Sports Science 19(12): 915-29.

94. Shiely, F., Hayes, K., MacDonncha, C. & Kelleher, C.C. (2004). Objectively Measured Physical Activity in Irish Adolescents Using Heart Rate Monitoring. Irish Journal of Medical Science, to appear.

95. McCarthy, S.N., Gibney, M.J., Flynn, A & Livingstone, M.B.E..; Irish Universities Nutrition Alliance (2002) Overweight, obesity and physical activity levels in Irish adults: evidence from the North/South Ireland Food Consumption Survey. Proceedings of the Nutrition Society; 61: 3-7.

96. Berkey CS, Rockett HR, Field AE, Gillman MW, Frazier AL, Camargo CA Jr, Colditz GA (2000) Activity, dietary intake, and weight changes in a longitudinal study of preadolescent and adolescent boys and girls. Pediatrics; 105(4):E56.

97. Wake M, Hesketh K, Waters E (2003) Television, computer use and body mass index in Australian primary school children. Journal of Paediatric and Child Health; 39 (2): 130-134.

98. Coon, K.A. & Tucker, K.L. (2002) Television and children's consumption patterns; a review of the literature. Minerva Pediatrica; 54(5):423-436.

99. Broadcasting Commission of Ireland (2003) Irish Children's TV Viewing Patterns. Children's Advertising Code Research into children's viewing patterns in Ireland. http://www.bci.ie/res.html

100. Todd, J. & Currie, D. (2003) Sedentary Behaviour. In Young People's Health in Context. Health Behaviour in School-Aged Children (HBSC) study: international report from the 2001/2002 survey. Currie et al. (Editors). WHO, Copenhagen, 2004. (www.hbsc.org).

101. Southern Health Board (2004) Our Children, their future, why weight? Survey Series & Literature Review on Childhood Obesity. Department of Public Health, Southern Health Board, December, 2004.

102. Saris, W.H.M., Blair, S.N., vanBaak, M.A., Eaton, S.B., Davies, P.S.N., DiPietro, L., Fogelholm, M., Rissanen, A., Scholler, D., Swinburn, B., Tremblay, A., Westerterp, K.R. & Wyatt, M. (2003) How much physical activity is enough to prevent unhealthy weight gain? Outcome of the IASO 1st STOCK conference and consensus statement. Obesity Reviews; 4:101-114.

103. Wadden, T.A. & Didie, E. (2003) What's in a name? Patients' preferred terms for describing obesity. Obesity Research; 11(9):1140-1146.

104. Gortmaker, S.L., Must, A., Perrin, J., Sobol A.M., Arthur, M. & Dietz, WH. (1993) Social and economic consequences of overweight in adolescence and young adulthood. New England Journal of Medicine; 329: 1008-1012.

105. Fabricatore A. & Wadden, A. (2004) Psychological aspects of obesity. Clinics in Dermatology;22: 332-337.

106. Puhl, R. & Brownell, K. D. (2001). Obesity, bias and discrimination. Obesity Research; 8: 788-805.

107. Puhl, R. & Brownell, K.D. (2003) Ways of coping with obesity stigma: review and conceptual analysis. Eating Behaviours; 4: 53-78.

108. Roehling, M.V. (1999) Weight based discrimination in employment: Psychological and legal aspects. Personality and Social Psychology Review; 52: 969-1017.

109. Baum C. & Ford, W.(2004) The wage effects of obesity: a longitudinal study. Health Economics; 13(9): 885.

110. Maiman, L.A., Wang, V.L., Becker, M.H., Finlay, J. & Simonson, M. (1979) Attitudes toward obesity and the obese among professionals. Journal of the American Dietetic Association;74:331–6.

111. Dietz, W. H. (1998). Health consequences of obesity in youth: childhood predictors of adult disease. Pediatrics 101: 518-525.

112. Hill, A. J., E. Draper, et al. (1994). A weight on children's minds: Body shape dissatisfaction at 9 years old. International Journal of Obesity 18: 383-389.

113. Wardle, J., C. Volz, et al. (1995). Social variation in attitudes to obesity in children. International Journal of Obesity 19: 562-569.

114. Falkner, N.H., Neumark-Sztainer, D., Story M., Jeffery R.W. & Resnick MD (2001) Social educational, and psychological correlates of weight status in adolescents Obesity Research; 9: 32-42.

115. Pearce, M., Boergers, J. & Prinstein M. (2002) Adolescent Obesity, Overt and Relational peer Victimization, and Romantic Relationships. Obesity Research; 10: 386-393.

116. Hellerstedt, W. L., Story, M. (1998). Adolescent satisfaction with postpartum contraception and body weight concerns. Journal of Adolescent Health 22: 446-452.

117. Anderson, P.M., Butsher, K.F. & Levine, P.B (2002) Maternal employment and overweight children. National Bureau of Economic Research. www.nber.org/papers/w/9247

118. Chou, S.Y., Grossman, M. & Saffer, H. (2002) An economic analysis of adult obesity: Results from the behavioural risk factor surveillance system. National Bureau of Economic Research. http://www.nber.org/papers/w9247

119. Lakdawalla, D. and Philipson, T. (2002) The growth of obesity and technological change: A theoretical and empirical examination. National Bureau of Economic Research; www.nber.org/papers/w8946

120. Cutler, D.M., Glaser, E.L. and Shapiro, J.M. (2003) Why have Americans become more obese? National Bureau of Economic Research; www.nber.org/papers/w9446

121. Cawley, J. (2004) An economic framework for understanding physical activity and eating behaviours. American Journal of Preventive Medicine; 27(3): S117-125.

122. Hill, J.O., Sallis, J.F. and Peters, J.C. (2004) Economic Analysis of eating and physical activity. A next step for research and policy change. American Journal of Preventive Medicine;27(3) :S111-S116.

123. National Roads Authority (2003) Road accident facts 2002.

124. Lobstein, T. (2004) 'Obesity and healthy eating- where did it all go wrong?'. Presentation given at HPU Conference on Tackling Obesity Together – Every Step Counts. Cavan, November, 2004.

125. National Audit Office (2001) Tackling Obesity in England: Report by the Comptroller and auditor general. Hcsso Session 200-2001. http://www.nao.org.uk/publications/nao_reports/00-01/0001220.pdf

126. Chief Medical Officer (2004) At least five a week: Evidence on the impact of physical activity and its relationship to health. London: Department of Health.

127. World Health Organisation (2004) Physical Activity http://www.who.int/dietphysicalactivity/publications/facts/pa/en/print.html 5th November 2004.WHO.

128. Central Statistics Office (2005) Consumer Price Index. December 2004.

129. Friel, S. & Conlon, C. (2004) Food Poverty and Policy. Combat Poverty Agency: Dublin.

130. Friel, S., Walsh, O. & McCarthy, D. (2004) Cost of Healthy Eating in the Republic of Ireland. Centre for Health Promotion Studies, NUI, Galway.

131. Women's Health Council (2004) Women, Disadvantage and Cardiovascular Disease: Policy Implications. Conference Proceedings, April, 2004. http://www.whc.ie/publications/ConfProc.pdf

132 Department of Health (2002) Annual Report of the Chief Medical Officer 2002.London: The Stationary Office.

133. International Diabetes Federation and International association for the study of Obesity " Diabetes and Obesity: Time to Act" International Diabetes Federation, 2004.

134. Pi-Sunyer Z., Becker D., Bouxhard C., Carleton R et al (1998).Clinical Guidelines on the Identification, Evaluation and Treatment of Overweight and Obesity in Adults: The Evidence Report. National Institute of Health No 98-4083.

135. Frick M H, Elo O, Haapa K, Heinonen O P, Heinsalmi P, Helo P, Huttunen J K, Kaitaniemi P, Koskinen P, Manninen V, Maenpaa H, Malkonen M, Manttari M, Norola S, Pasternack A, Pikkarainen J, Romo M. Sjöblom T & Nikkilä E A (1987). Helsinki Heart Study: primary-prevention trial with gemfibrozil in middle-aged men with dyslipidemia. Safety of treatment, changes in risk factors, and incidence of coronary heart disease. New England Journal of Medicine 317:1237-45

136. (The) Lipid Research Clinics Coronary Primary Prevention Trial results. I.(1984) Reduction in incidence of coronary heart disease. Journal of the American Medical Association, 20;251(3):351-64.

137. McPherson, K Steel, C M & Dixon J M. ABC of breast diseases: Breast cancer epidemiology, risk factors, and genetics. British Medical Journal; 321: 624 - 628.

138. Huang, Z., Hankinson, S. E., Colditz, G. A., Stampfer, M. J., Hunter, D. J., Manson, J. E., Hennekens, C. H., Rosner, B., Speizer, F. E., Willett, W. C. (1997). Dual effects of weight and weight gain on breast cancer risk. Journal of the American Medical Association 278: 1407-1411.

139. Stoll, B. A. (1998). Teenage obesity in relation to breast cancer risk. International Journal of Obesity 22: 1035-1040.

140. Strauss R. (2000) Childhood obesity and self-esteem. Pediatrics, Vol 105.

141. Kimm, S., Barton, B.A., Berhane, K. & Ross J. (1997) Self esteem and adiposity in Black and White girls: The NHLBI Growth and Health Study. Annals of Epidemiology; 7:550-560.

142. Wadden, T.A., Steen, S.N., Wingate, B.J. & Foster, G.D. (1996) Psychosocial consequences of weight reduction: how much weight loss is enough? America Journal of Clinical Nutrition;63: 461S-465S.

143. Germov J., Williams L.(1996) The Epidemic of Dieting Women: The need for a Sociological Approach to Food and Nutrition. Appetite; 27: 97-108.

144. Carpenter K.M., Heisin, D.S. Allison, D.B., et al (2000) Relationships between obesity and DSM-IV major depressive disorder, suicide ideation, and suicide attempts: Results from a

general population study. American Journal of Public Health; 90: 251-257.
145. Istvan J., Zavela K. & Weidner G. (1992) Body weight and psychological distress in NHANES. International Journal of Obesity; 16:999-1003.

146. Onyike, C.U., Crum, R.M., Lee, H.B., Lyketsos, C.G. & Eaton, W.W (2003) Is obesity associated with major Depression ?- Results from the Third National Health and Nutrition Examination Survey. American Journal of Epidemiology; 158:12 1139.

147. Must, A., P. F. Jacques, et al. (1992). Longterm morbidity and mortality of overweight adolescents: A follow-up of the Harvard Growth Study of 1922 to 1935. New England Journal of Medicine 327(19): 1350 - 1355.

148. Janssen, I., Craig, W., Boyce, W., Pickett, W., (2004) Associations between overweight and obesity with bullying behaviour in School- aged children. Paediatrics 113: 1187-1194.

149. U.S Dept of Health and Human Services (USDHHS). Physical activity and health. A report of the surgeon general. Atlanta, GA: US Department of Health and Human Services; Centres for disease control and prevention.

150.Poulsen A. & Ziviani J. (2004) Health enhancing physical activity: Factors influencing engagement patterns in children. Australian Occupational Therapy Journal 51, 69-79.

151. Wei, M., Kampert, J.B., Barlow, C.E., Nichaman, M.Z., Gibbons, L.W., Paffenbarger, R.S. Jr., Blair. S.N. (1999) Relationship between low cardiorespiratory fitness and mortality in normal-weight, overweight, and obese men. Journal of the American Medical Association; 282(16):1547-53.

152. European Heart Health Initiative (2001) Children & Young People- the importance of Physical activity. Brussels.

153. U.S. Department of Health and Human Services (USDHHS). The Surgeon General's call to action to prevent and decrease overweight and obesity. U.S. GPO, Washington, 2001.

154. Swinburn, B. & Egger, G. (2002) Prevention strategies against weight gain and obesity. Obesity Reviews; 3: 289-301.

155. Macmillian Dictionary (2002) http://www.macmillandictionary.com/New-Words/031121-obesogenic.htm

156. Sohun, R., & MacDonncha, C. (2001). The Impact of Physical Education Provision in Post-Primary Schools on Physical Activity, Physical Fitness and Psychological Parameters in a Cohort of Irish Adolescents. Unpublished Masters Thesis, Department of Physical Education and Sport Sciences, University of Limerick, Ireland.

157. Physical Activity Task Force. (2002) Let's Make Scotland More Active. The Stationary Office, Edinburgh.

158. Trost SG, Kerr LM, Ward DS, Pate RR. (2001) Physical activity and determinants of physical activity in obese and non-obese children. International Journal of Obesity. 25, 822-829.

159. Gordon-Larsen P, Nelson M, Popkin B. (2004) Longitudinal Physical Acitivy and Sedentary Behavior Trends Adolecence to Adulthood. American Journal of Preventive Medicine; 27 (4).

160. Plotnikoff, R.C., Mayhew, A., Birkett, N., Loucaides, C.A., Fodor, G.(2004) Age, gender, and urban-rural differences in the correlates of physical activity. Preventive Medicine;39(6):1115-1125.

161. Sallis, J. & Owen, N. Physical activity and behavioural medicine. Thousand oaks, CA: Sage publishers. 1999.

162. Sallis, J.F., Kraft, K. & Linton, L.S. (2002) How the environment shapes physical activity: a transdisciplinary research agenda. American Journal of Preventive Medicine; 22(3): 208.

163. Ministry of Health, New Zealand (2003) DHB Toolkit: Physical activity – to increase physical activity. Ministry of Health, Wellington. http://www.newhealth.govt.nz/toolkits/physical/PhysicalActivityToolkit03.pdf

164. Mela, D.J. (2001) Determinants of food choice: Relationships with Obesity and Weight Control. Obesity Research; 9(4): 249S-255S.

165. Sustain (1993). Get cooking! London: National Food Alliance, Department of Health and BBC Good Food.

166. Lang T, Caraher M Dixon P & Carr-Hill R (1999) Cooking Skills and Health: Inequalities in Health. London: Health Education Authority. http://www.hda-online.org.uk/Documents/cooking_skills_health.pdf

167. Hawkes, C. (2004) Marketing Food to Children: the global regulatory environment. World Health Organisation: Geneva.

168. Goldberg. J.P. & Hellwig, J.P. (1997) Nutrition Research in the media: The challenge facing scientists. Journal of American College of Nutrition, 16(6): 544 550.

169. Breakdown of Advertising and Share Expenditure – BASE (2003) Full Year Report http://www.iapi.com/base/report1203.pdf

170. Checkout Ireland (2003) Top 100 Brands 2003 www.checkout.ie/Top100.asp

171. Food Commission, UK (2003) Broadcasting bad health: Why food marketing to children needs to be controlled. A report by the International Association of Consumer Food Organizations for the World Health Organization consultation on a global strategy for diet and health.
http://www.foodcomm.org.uk/Broadcasting_bad_health.pdf

172. Hastings, G., Stead, M., McDermott, L., Forsyth, A., MacKintosh, A.M., Rayner, M., Godfrey, C., Caraher, M. & Angus, K. (2003) Review of the research on the effects of food promotion to children. Final Report. Food Standards Agency.
www.foodstandards.gov.uk/multimedia/pdfs/foodpromotiontochildren1.pdf

173. Borzekowski, D.L. & Robinson, T.N. (2001) The 30-second effect: An experiment revealing the impact of television commercials on food preferences of preschoolers. Journal of the American Dietetic Association; 101(1):42-46.

174. Robinson, T.N., Chen, H.L. & Killen, J.D. (1998) Television and Music Video Exposure and risk of adolescent alcohol use. Paediatrics; 102 (5): E54.

175. Valkenburg PM. (2000) Media and youth consumerism. Journal of Adolescent Health. 27 S, 52–56.

176. Byrd-Bredbenner, C. & Grasso, D. (2000) Health, medicine, and food messages in television commercials during 1992 and 1998. Journal of School Health; 70(2): 61-65.

177. Consumers International (2002) A spoonful of sugar: television food advertising aimed at children: an international comparative survey.
www.consumersinternational.org/campaigns/tvads/index.html

178. Oliver, J.E. & Lee, T. (2002) Public opinion and the politics of America's Obesity epidemic. KSG Working Paper series, Harvard University.

179. Tillotson, J.E. (2004) America's Obesity: Conflicting public policies, industrial economic development, and unintended human consequences. Annual Reviews of Nutrition; 24:617-643.

180. Nestle, M. & Jacobson, M.F. (2000) Halting the obesity epidemic: A public health policy approach. Public Health Reports; 115: 12-24.

181. UK Public Health Association and Faculty of Public Health Medicine (2003) Joint Submission to the House of Commons Health Committee Inquiry on Obesity.
http://www.fphm.org.uk/Consultations/Responses_to_consultations/2003/April/obesity_inquiry_evidence_300403.pdf

182. Leicester, A. & Windmeijer, F. (2004) The 'Fat Tax': Economic Incentives to reduce obesity. Institute for Fiscal Studies Briefing Note No.49; London.

183. Sallis J, Bauman A, Pratt M. (1998) Environmental and Policy Interventions to Promote Physical Activity. American Journal Preventive Med; 15 (4):379-397.

184. Sallis, J., Johnson,M., Calfas, K.,Caparosa, S., & Nichols, J., (1997) Assessing the physical environmental variables that may influence physical activity. Research quarterly for Exercise and Sport, 68, 345-351.

185. Humpel, N., Owen, N. and Leslie, E. (2002) Environmental factors associated with adults' participation in physical activity: a review. American Journal Preventive Medicine; 22:188–199.

186. Gordon-Larsen P, McMurray R.G, Popkin. B (2000) Determinants of Adolescent Physical Activity and Inactivity Patterns. Pediatrics Vol. 105 No. 6.

187. Sallis, J.F., Hovell, M.F., Hofstetter, C.R., Faucher, P., Elder, J.P., Blanchard, J., Caspersen, C.J., Powell, K.E., Christenson, G.M.(1989) A multivariate study of determinants of vigorous exercise in a community sample. Preventive Medicine;18(1):20-34.

188. Sallis, J.F., Nader, P.R., Broyles, S.L., Berry, C.C. et al (1993) Correlates of physical activity at home in Mexican-American and Anglo-American preschool children. Health Psychology; 12(5) 390-398.

189. Foster C, Hillsdon M. (2004) Changing the environment to promote health-enhancing physical activity. Journal of Sports Science;22(8):755-69.

190. Campbell, K., Waters, E., O'Meara, S., Kelly, S. & Summerbell, C. Interventions for preventing obesity in children (Cochrane Review). The Cochrane Library, Issue 1, 2004. Chichester, UK: John Wiley & Sons, Ltd.

191. Douketis, J.D., Feightner, J.W., Attia, J., Feldmen, W.F. with the Canadian TaskForce on Preventive Health Care. (1999) Periodic health examination, 1999: Update 1.

192. Patton, G. C., R. Selzer, et al. (1999). Onset of adolescent eating disorders: population-based cohort study over 3 years. British Medical Journal 318: 765-768.

193. Dietz, W. H. and R. Hartung (1985). Changes in height velocity of obese pre-adolescents during weight reduction. American Journal of Diseases of Childhood 139: 705-707.

194. Epstein, L. H., M. D. Myers, et al. (1998). Treatment of pediatric obesity. Pediatrics 101: 554-570.

195. Flynn, M.A.T. (2003) Community Prevention of Obesity in Canada: The technical document Calgary Health Region.

196. Puska, P., Vartiainen, E., Tuomilehto, J., Salomaa, V. & Nissinen A. (1998) Changes in premature deaths in Finland; successful long-term prevention of cardiovascular diseases. Bulletin of the World Health Organisation, 1998, 76 (4):419-425.

197. Health Canada (2001). The population health template: Key elements and actions that define a population health approach, draft July, Health Canada Population and Public health Branch, Strategic Policy directorate. Ottawa.

198. Orleans, C. T. (2000). Promoting the maintenance of health behavior change:recommendations for the next generation of research and practice. Health Psychology 19(1Supplement): S76-S83.

199. Egger, G. and B. Swinburn (1997). An "ecological" approach to the obesity pandemic. British Medical Journal of Public Health 315((7106)): 477 - 480.

200. Kumanyika, S. K. (2001). Minisymposium on Obesity: Overview and Some Strategic Considerations. Annual Review Public Health 22: 293 - 308.

201. Ebbeling, C.B., Rawlak, D.B. & Ludwig, D.S. (2002) Childhood obesity: public-health crisis, common sense sure. The Lancet; 360: 473-482.

202. Egger, G., Swinburn, B. & Rossner, S. (2003) Dusting off the epidemiological triad: Could it work with obesity? Obesity Reviews; 4:115-119.

203. NHS CRD (Centre for Reviews and Dissemination) (1997).A systematic review of the interventions for the prevention and treatment of obesity, and the maintenance of weight loss. CRD Report 10, University of York.

204. Hardeman, W., Griffin, S., Johnston, M., Kinmonth, A.L. & Wareham, N.J.(2000) Intervention to prevent weight gain: a systematic review of psychological models and behaviour change methods. International Journal of Obesity; 24: 131-143.

205. NHS CRD (Centre for Reviews and Dissemination) (2002).The prevention and treatment of childhood obesity.Effective Health Care 7 (6)

206. Mulvihill, C & Quigley, R. (2003) The management of obesity and overweight: An analysis of reviews of diet, physical activity and behavioural approaches. Evidence Briefing. Health Development Agency: London. www.had.nhs.uk/documents/obesity_evidence_briefing.pdf.

207. Hillsdon, M., Foster, C., Naidoo, B & Crombie, H. (2004) The effectiveness of public health interventions for increasing physical activity among adults. Evidence briefing. www.nhs.hda/evidence

208. Robinson, T.N. (2001) Television viewing and childhood obesity. Paediatric Clinic of North America; 48(4):1017-1025.

209. Sallis, J.F., Alcaraz, J.E., McKenzie, T.L., Hovell, M.F., Kolody, B., Nader, P.R. (1992) Parental behavior in relation to physical activity and fitness in 9-year-old children. American Journal of Diseases of Children;146(11):1383-1388.

210. Serdula, M. K., A. H. Mokdad, et al. (1999). Prevalence of attempting weight loss and strategies for controlling weight. Journal of the American Medical Association 282(14).

211. Klein S, Sheard NF, Pi-Sunyer X, Daly A, Wylie-Rosett J, Kulkarni K, Clark NG; American Diabetes Association; North American Association for the Study of Obesity; American Society for Clinical Nutrition (2004) Weight management through lifestyle modification for the prevention and management of type 2 diabetes: rationale and strategies. A statement of the American Diabetes Association, the North American Association for the Study of Obesity, and the American Society for Clinical Nutrition. American Journal of Clinical Nutrition 80(2):257-263.

212. Lee, C. D., Blair, S. N., Jackson, A. S. (1999). Cardiorespiratory fitness, body composition and al cause cardiovascular disease mortality in men. American Journal of Nutrition 69: 373-380.

213. Yancy, W.S. Jr, Olsen, M.K., Guyton, J.R., Bakst, R.P., Westman, E.C. (2004) Low-carbohydrate, ketogenic diet versus a low-fat diet to treat obesity and hyperlipidemia: a randomized, controlled trial. Annals of Internal Medicine;140(10):769-77.

214. Woodward-Lopez, G. (2004) Framework for Obesity Prevention. Centre for Weight and Health, University of California. Personal Communication.

215. Friel, S., Kelleher, C., Campbell, P. & Nolan, G. (1999) Evaluation of the Nutrition Education at Primary School (NEAPS) programme. Public Health Nutrition; 2(4): 549-555.

216. Lowe, C.F., Horne, P.J., Tapper, K An evaluation of the Food Dude Healthy Eating Programme in Ireland. Bord Glas. Dublin, 2004.

217. Johnson, Z., Molloy, B., Scallan, E., Fitzpatrick, P., Rooney, B., Keegan, T,, Byrne, P. (2000) Community Mothers Programme--seven year follow-up of a randomized controlled trial of non-professional intervention in parenting. Journal of Public Health Medicine; 22(3):337-42.

218. Australian National Health and Medical Research Council -ANHMRC (2003) Clincial practice guidelines for the management of overweight and obesity. www.obesityguidelines.gov.au.

219. European Association for the Study of Obesity - EASO (2004) Management of Obesity in adults: Project for European Primary Care. International Journal of Obesity; 28: 226S-231S.

220. National Institutes of Health (NIH), National Heart, Lung and Blood Institute (NHLBI). The Practical Guide: Identification, evaluation, and treatment of overweight and obesity in adults. HHS, Public Health Services (PHS); 2000. http://www.nhlbi.nih.gov/guidelines/obesity/ob_home.htm

221a. National Obesity Forum - NOF. (2004) Guidelines on Management of Adult Obesity and Overweight in Primary Care. www.nationalobesityforum.org.uk

221b. National Obesity Forum NOF- NOF (2004). Guidelines on Management of Children Obesity and Overweight in Primary Care. www.nationalobesityforum.org.uk

221c. National Obesity Forum- NOF (2004). Pharmacotherapy Guidelines for Obesity Management in Adults. www.nationalobesityforum.org.uk

222. Scottish Intercollegiate Guidelines Network –SIGN (1996) Obesity in Scotland: Integrating Prevention with Weight Management. A National Clinical Guideline recommended for use in Scotland – Pilot Edition. www.sign.ac.uk/guidelines/published/

223. Scottish Intercollegiate Guidelines Network- SIGN (2003) Management of obesity in children and young people. www.sign.ac.uk/guidelines/published/

224. Fernandez, A.Z., Demaria, E.J., Tichansky, D.S., Kellum, J.M., Wolfe, L.G., Meador, J. & Sugerman, H.J. (2004) Multivariate Analysis of Risk Factors for Death Following Gastric Bypass for Treatment of Morbid Obesity. Annals of Surgery. 239(5):698-703.

225. Chestnutt, I.G. & Ashraf, F.J. (2002) Television advertising of foodstuffs potentially detrimental to oral health – a content analysis and comparison of children's and primetime broadcasts. Community Dental Health; 19: 86-89.

226. Gillman, M.W., Rifas-Shiman, S.L., Frazier, A.L., Rockett, H.R.H, Camargo, C.A., Field, A.E, Berkey, C.S. & Colditz, G.A. (2000) Family dinner and diet quality among older children and adolescents. Archives of Family Medicine; 9: 235-240.

Glossary of Terms

Adiposity – the property or state of being fat.

Aerobic fitness – increases the amount of oxygen that is delivered to your muscles, which allows them to work longer.

Algorithm – A step-by-step protocol, as for management of health care problems.

Atherogenic – cause the formation of abnormal fat deposits (plaques) on the walls of arteries.

Calorie – A calorie is a unit that measures energy. Calories come from four sources: carbohydrate, fat, protein and alcohol.

Discretionary Calories – Calories that remain within a person's caloric allowance after all nutrient recommendations are met.

Energy Density is defined as the amount of energy per unit weight of food. It can be listed as kcal/g or, as kJ/100g.

Epidemiology – the study of the causes, distribution, and control of disease in populations.

Fatty acids – the major parts of fat. Depending on their chemical structure, fatty acids are classified as either saturated or unsaturated. There are two types of unsaturated fats: monounsaturated and polyunsaturated.

Fibrinogen – A protein in the blood plasma that is essential for the coagulation of blood.

Glycaemic Response – A measure of how quickly and how high specific foods raise blood sugar level (i.e converted from carbohydrates in food to glucose in the blood).

Glycaemic index – The Glycaemic Index is a numerical Index that ranks carbohydrates based on their rate of glycaemic response (Glycaemic Index uses a scale of 0 to 100, with higher values given to foods that cause the most rapid rise in blood sugar. Pure glucose serves as a reference point, and is given a Glycaemic Index (GI) of 100.

Health Promoting School – aims at achieving healthy lifestyles for the total school population by developing supportive environments conducive to the promotion of health. It offers opportunities for, and requires commitments to, the provision of a safe and health-enhancing social and physical environment (WHO, 1993).

Health proofing – examining public policies to ensure they protect public health.

High-density lipoprotein (HDL), - sometimes referred to as "good" or protective cholesterol, because they carry cholesterol away from the arteries to the liver to be excreted from the body.

Hypokinetic diseases – diseases which relate to low movement or activity.

Life skills – the ability to cope with stresses and challenges of daily life, especially skills in communication and literacy, decision-making, occupational requirements, problem-solving, time management and planning.

Lifestyle – The unique and personal customs or habits of an individual. It is their active adaptation to the social environment which develops as a product of need for integration and socialisation. It includes; social use of substances such as alcohol and tobacco, dietary habits, exercise, etc., all of which have important implications for health.

Lipoprotein – protein molecules in the blood transport cholesterol through the blood vessels. The amounts and types of lipoproteins are an important indicator of your heart disease risk.

Low-density lipoprotein (LDL) – sometimes referred to as "bad" cholesterol, because an excess of cholesterol carried by them can lead to the build up of plaque in the arteries. LDLs are not found in food, only in the body.

Metabolic regulation – control of the biochemical processes involved in life.

Obesogenic – developed from a blend of the word obese and, by analogy with terms like *carcinogenic* (causing cancer), -genic as a suffix meaning 'tending to create'.

Passive over-consumption – unintentional over-eating or accidentally eating more calories than needed.

Percentile – value on a scale of one hundred that indicates the percent of a distribution that is equal to or below it.

Precautionary Principle – the ethical principle that if the consequences of an action are unknown but are judged to have a high risk of being negative from an ethical point of view, then it is better not to carry out the action rather than risk the uncertain, but possibly very negative, consequences.

Prevalence – the percentage of a population that is affected with a particular condition at a given time.

Relative Risk – a measure of how much a particular risk factor influences the risk of a specified outcome in someone with the risk factor compared to someone without.

Work-Life Balance – Meaningful daily achievement and enjoyment in work, family, friends and self.

List of Figures

Appendices

APPENDIX A

Membership of the National Taskforce on Obesity:

Mr John Treacy	Irish Sports Council (Chair)
Mr Chris Fitzgerald	Department of Health and Children
Mr Ciarán Fitzgerald	Food & Drink Industry Ireland, IBEC
Dr Brian Gaffney	Health Promotion Agency for Northern Ireland
Ms Jacky Jones	Health Service Executive, Western Area
Ms Siobhan Julian	Irish Nutrition & Dietetic Institute
Prof Cecily Kelleher	University College Dublin
Ms Marie Kennedy	National Children's Office
Dr Marie Laffoy	Health Service Executive Eastern Regional Area
Ms Fiona Lalor	Food & Drink Industry Ireland, IBEC
Mr Michael Maloney	An Bord Glas
Ms. Maureen Mulvihill	Irish Heart Foundation
Ms Ursula O'Dwyer	Department of Health and Children
Mr Donal O'Gorman	Exercise & Sports Science Association of Ireland
Dr John Mark O'Riordan	Irish College of General Practitioners
Dr Donal O'Shea	St. Colmcilles Hospital, Loughlinstown: St. Vincents University Hospital
Dr Thomas Quigley	safefood the Food Safety Promotion Board
Mr Alan Reilly	Food Safety Authority of Ireland
Dr Helen Whelton	Oral Health Services Research Centre
Dr Jane Wilde	Institute of Public Health

Secretariat:

Ms Oilbhe O'Donoghue	Department of Health and Children (secretary)
Ms. Debbie Corradino	National Nutrition Surveillance Centre
Mr Brian Dowling (replaced Mr. Brian Brogan)	Department of Health and Children
Dr Deirdre Mulholland	Health Service Executive Eastern Regional Area
Ms Celine Murrin	National Nutrition Surveillance Centre
Ms Geraldine Nolan	National Nutrition Surveillance Centre
Dr Frances Shiely	National Nutrition Surveillance Centre

Detection and Treatment Sub-committee:

Dr Donal O'Shea	St. Colmcilles Hospital, Loughlinstown (Chair)
Ms Celine Murrin	National Nutrition Surveillance Centre (Secretary)
Ms Siobhan Julian	Irish Nutrition & Dietetic Institute
Dr Marie Laffoy	Health Service Executive Eastern Regional Area
Dr. Deirdre Mulholland	Health Service Executive Eastern Regional Area
Mr Donal O'Gorman	Exercise & Sports Science Association of Ireland
Dr John Mark O'Riordan	Irish College of General Practitioners
Mr John Treacy	Irish Sports Council

Public Sector Sub-committee:

Prof Cecily Kelleher	University College Dublin (Chair)
Ms Oilbhe O'Donoghue	Department of Health and Children (Secretary)
Dr Thomas Quigley	safefood the Food Safety Promotion Board
Ms Marie Kennedy	National Children's Office
Ms Ursula O'Dwyer	Department of Health and Children
Ms. Maureen Mulvihill	Irish Heart Foundation
Dr Brian Gaffney	Health Promotion Agency for Northern Ireland
Mr Alan Reilly	Food Safety Authority of Ireland
Mr John Treacy	Irish Sports Council
Mr Chris Fitzgerald	Department of Health and Children
Dr Helen Whelton	Oral Health Services Research Centre

Private Sector Sub-committee:

Ms Fiona Lalor	Food & Drink Industry Ireland, IBEC (Chair)
Mr Michael Maloney	An Bord Glas
Dr Marie Laffoy	Health Service Executive Eastern Regional Area
Mr Alan Reilly	Food Safety Authority of Ireland
Ms Jacky Jones	Health Service Executive, Western Area
Mr Donal O'Gorman	Exercise & Sports Science Association of Ireland
Mr Chris Fitzgerald	Department of Health and Children
Mr John Treacy	Irish Sports Council

Editorial Sub-committee:

Mr Chris Fitzgerald	Department of Health and Children (Chair)
Mr Brian Dowling	Department of Health and Children
Prof Cecily Kelleher	University College Dublin
Dr Marie Laffoy	Health Service Executive Eastern Regional Area
Dr Deirdre Mulholland	Health Service Executive Eastern Regional Area
Ms Celine Murrin	National Nutrition Surveillance Centre
Ms Oilbhe O'Donoghue	Department of Health and Children
Mr John Treacy	Irish Sports Council

APPENDIX B

Submissions

In addition to receiving 104 submissions from individuals, the National Taskforce on Obesity received submissions from the following:

Abbott Laboratories
Adelaide and Meath Hospital
Adelaide and Meath Hospital, Cardiology Department
Association of Lactation Consultants in Ireland (ALCI)
Association of Secondary Teachers Ireland
Astro Park
Badminton Union of Ireland
Beverage Council of Ireland
Bodywhys
Bord Bia
Burger King
BWG Foods Limited
Cadbury
Cafeslim
Cantrell and Cochrane Group
Catering Management Association
Catholic Youth Care
Céifin Centre
Centre for Early Childhood Development & Education
Childcare Directory
Children's Rights Alliance
Children's University Hospital
Chocolate, Confectionery and Biscuit Council of Ireland
Clare County Council
Coca-Cola
Combat Poverty Agency
Community Dietitian Managers
Consumer Association of Ireland
County Cork Sports Partnership
Deaforward
Department of Agriculture and Food
Department of Arts, Sport and Tourism
Department of Education & Science
Department of Finance
Department of Health, Social Services and Public Safety, Northern Ireland
Diabetes Federation of Ireland
Domino's Pizza
Dublin City Council
Dublin City University, Centre for Sport Science and Health
Dublin Cycling Campaign
Dublin Institute of Technology, Human Nutrition and Dietetics
East Coast Area Health Board, Health Promotion Department
Eastern Regional Health Authority, Public Health Medicine

Economic and Social Research Institute
Eddie Rockets
Edendum Fine Catering
EU Coaching
European Institute of Womens Health
European Year of Education through Sport
Exercise and Sport Science Assocociation of Ireland
Expo Exhibitions Limited
Fit 'n' Fun
Focus Ireland
Food Safety Authority of Ireland
Football Association of Ireland
Fyffes
Gaelic Athletic Association
Galway City Community Forum
Galway Cycling Campaign
Glanbia
Green Party
Health Boards Executive, Programme of Action for Children
Health Research Board
Heinz
Herbalife
IMAC Academy of Tai Chi
INAMED
Institute of Advertising Practitioners in Ireland and the Association of Advertisers in Ireland
Institute of Community Health Nursing
Institute of Irish Medical Herbalists
Institute of Leisure and Amenity Management
Irish Association for Councelling and Psychotherapy
Irish Association of Dance Teachers
Irish Bread Bakers Association
Irish Business and Employers Confederation
Irish Cancer Society
Irish College of General Practitioners
Irish College of Psychiatrists
Irish Dairy Industries Association
Irish Farmers Association
Irish Health Trade Association
Irish Heart Foundation
Irish Ladies' Golf Union
Irish Medicines Board
Irish Mental Patients' Educational and Representative Organisation
Irish National Teachers Organisation
Irish Nutrition and Dietetic Institute
Irish Osteoporosis Society
Irish Pharamaceutical Union
Irish Sailing Association
Irish Society of Chartered Physiotherapists
Irish Sports Council

Irish Sugar
Johnson and Johnson Medical
Keep Ireland Open
Kenny Marketing
Kerry County Development Board
Kerry Local Sports Partnership
La Leche League
Limerick City Sports Partnership
Limerick Local Sports Partnership
Marino Therapy Centre
Mary Immaculate College
McDonalds
Meath Local Sports Partnerships
Midland Health Board, Department of Public Health and Planning
Mid-western Health Board
Mid-western Health Board, Maternity Hospital
Motivation Weight Control Clinics
Mountaineering Council of Ireland
Musgrave SuperValu•Centra
Natioanl University of Ireland, Galway
National Association for Deaf People
National Association for People with an Intellectual Disability
National Certificate in Exercise and Fitness
National Children's Hospital (AMNCH)
National Children's Office
National Council on Ageing and Older People
National Dairy Council
National Disability Authority
National Heart Alliance
National Paediatric Nursing Advisory Forum
National Parents Council, Primary
Nestle
North Eeastern Health Board, Regional and Community Services
North Tipperary County Council
North Western Health Board
North Western Health Board, Public Health Department
Northern Area Health Board, Community and Primary Care Services
Nurture Point
Occupational Health Nurses Association of Ireland
O'Donovan's Pharmacy, Cork
Offaly County Council
Oral Health Promotion Research Group, Irish Link
Owens DDB
PepsiCo International
Pfizer
Physical Education Association of Ireland
Playball
Psychological Society of Ireland
Rangelands Foods Limited

Redbranch Human Performance
Restaurants Association of Ireland
Retail, Grocery, Dairy and Allied Trades' Association
Roche
Roscommon County Council
Roscommon Sports Partnership
Royal College of Surgeons in Ireland, Faculty of Sports and Exercise Medicine
Rutland Centre
safefood, the Food Safety Promotion Board
Scoil Phobail Sliabh Luachra
Senator Mary Henry
Siobhán Collins, Management Consultant
Sligo Sport and Recreation
Snack Food Association of Ireland
Social, Personal and Health Education, Support Service, Post Primary
Society of Chief and Principal Dental Surgeons
South Dublin County Council
South Eastern Health Board
South Eastern Health Board, Public Health Medicine
Southern Health Board, Health Promotion Department
Southern Health Board, Public Health Medicine
Southern Health Board, Public Health Nursing
Special Olympics Ireland
Sportsfit Software
St. Angela's College, Home Economics Department
St. Vincent's University Hospital
St. Vincents University Hospital, Department of Preventative Medicine and Health Promotion
Statoil
Storm marketing and design
Stretch-n-grow
Superquinn
Sutton to Sandycove Cycleway and Promenade Campaign
Swim Ireland
Tayto
Teagasc
Tesco Ireland
Tralee Institute of Technology, Health and Leisure Department
Trinity College Dublin
Trinity College Dublin, Department of Paediatrics
Trinity College Dublin, School of Nursing and Midwifery Studies
Trinity College Dublin, Unit of Nutrition and Dietetic Studies
Unilever Bestfoods Ireland
University College Cork, Deartment of Human Resources
University College Cork, Department of Epidemiology and Public Health
University College Cork, Occupational Therapy
University College Dublin
University of Limerick, Department of Physical Education and Sport Sciences
VHI Healthcare
Waterford City Council

Waterford Corporation
Waterford Institute of Technology
Waterford Sports Partnerships
Weight Watchers
Western Health Board, Corporate and Public Affairs
Western Health Board, Department of Public Health
Wexford County Council
White Mountain Dreams
Wicklow County Council
Women's Health Council

Presentations

In order to inform members of the Taskforce on the prevalence of obesity and the factors associated with it, presentations were made to the Taskforce at the second plenary meeting as follows;

- Obesity; the scale, causes and identifying solutions
  Ms. Celine Murrin, Researcher, National Nutrition Surveillance Centre, UCD
- The role of nutrition in addressing obesity
  Ms. Ursula O'Dwyer, Consultant Dietitian, Deparment of Health and Children
- The role of physical activity in addressing obesity
  Dr. Donal O'Gorman, Department of Sports Science and Health, DCU
- Detecting and treating obesity in clinical practice
  Dr. Donal O'Shea, Consultant Endocrinologist, Loughlinstown Hospital

Additionally, the following made expert presentations to the Taskforce, during the course of its work:

- Dr. Tim Lobstein — International Taskforce on Obesity
- Mr. Peter Smith — Irish Sports Council
- Mr. Ciarán Fitzgerald — Food & Drink Industry Ireland, IBEC
- Prof. Fergus Lowe — University of Wales, Bangor
- Dr. Mary Flynn — Calgary Health Region and Universities of Calgary and Alberta, Canada.

Acknowledgements

The National Taskforce on Obesity would like to acknowledge Joe Durkan, Economist, Geary Institute, UCD, for his contribution to drafting this document.

APPENDIX C

The following criteria are used to describe the strength of evidence in this report. They are based on the criteria used by the World Cancer Research Fund (1997) but were modified by the Joint WHO/FAO Expert Consultation to include the results of controlled trials where relevant and available. In addition, consistent evidence on community and environmental factors which lead to behaviour changes and thereby modify risks was taken into account in categorizing risks. This applies particularly to the complex interaction between environmental factors that affect excess weight gain, a risk factor which the Consultation recognized as contributing to many of the problems being considered.

Convincing evidence. Evidence based on epidemiological studies showing consistent associations between exposure and disease, with little or no evidence to the contrary. The available evidence is based on a substantial number of studies including prospective observational studies and where relevant, randomized controlled trials of sufficient size, duration and quality showing consistent effects. The association should be biologically plausible.

Probable evidence. Evidence based on epidemiological studies showing fairly consistent associations between exposure and disease, but where there are perceived shortcomings in the available evidence or some evidence to the contrary, which precludes a more definite judgement. Shortcomings in the evidence may be any of the following: insufficient duration of trials (or studies); insufficient trials (or studies) available; inadequate sample sizes; incomplete follow-up. Laboratory evidence is usually supportive.Again, the association should be biologically plausible.

Possible evidence. Evidence based mainly on findings from case--control and cross-sectional studies. Insufficient randomized controlled trials, observational studies or non-randomized controlled trials are available. Evidence based on non-epidemiological studies, such as clinical and laboratory investigations, is supportive. More trials are required to support the tentative associations, which should also be biologically plausible.

Insufficient evidence. Evidence based on findings of a few studies which are suggestive, but are insufficient to establish an association between exposure and disease. Limited or no evidence is available from randomized controlled trials. More well designed research is required to support the tentative associations.

APPENDIX D

The management of obesity and overweight
An analysis of reviews of diet, physical activity and behavioural approaches
(Mulvihill & Quigley, 2003)NHS, Health Development Agency

Treatment of obesity and overweight in children and adolescents
Three systematic reviews investigated the treatment of obesity and overweight in children (NHS CRD, 1997; NHS CRD, 2002; LeMura and Maziekas, 2002).
There is evidence:

- That targeting parents and children together (familybased interventions, involving at least one parent with physical activity and health promotion) is effective in treating obesity and overweight in children
- To support the use of multi-faceted family-based behaviour modification programmes, where parents take primary responsibility for behaviour change, in the treatment of obesity and overweight in primary schoolchildren. The programmes comprised diet,exercise, reducing sedentary behaviour and lifestyle counselling, with training in child management, parenting and communication skills
- To support the use of laboratory-based exercise programmes in the treatment of childhood obesity.These programmes consisted of walking, jogging, cycle ergometry, high-repetition resistance exercise and combinations within a laboratory setting, as opposed to free-living lifestyle activity interventions.

Currently, there is limited* evidence that behaviour modification programmes with no parental involvementare effective in the treatment of childhood obesity and overweight. These programmes included a reduced calorie diet and an exercise programme, combined with cognitive-behavioural 'obesity-training', or muscle relaxation training.

Currently, there is a lack of evidence for family-based behaviour modification programmes for the treatment of childhood obesity. These programmes included behaviour modification, dietary and exercise education with a mix of sessions involving the child, parent(s) and, in some cases,the entire family. At present there is insufficient evidence
to recommend any specific programme.

Treatment of obesity and overweight in adults
Diet
There is a large quantity of evidence on the effectiveness of dietary interventions for the treatment of obesity and overweight. The NHS CRD (1997), the National Heart,
Lung and Blood Institute (NIH, 1998), Astrup et al. (2000), and Pirozzo et al. (2002) examined this topic.The most common dietary interventions are low calorie diets, very low calorie diets and low fat diets.

There is evidence to:

- Support the effectiveness of low calorie diets (1,000-1,500 kilocalories per day)
- Suggest that clinically prescribed very low calorie diets (400-500 kilocalories per day) are more effective for acute weight loss than low calorie diets. However, there is conflicting evidence regarding the relative effectiveness of very low calorie diets versus low calorie diets over the long term (greater than one year)

- Support the effectiveness of low fat and low energy diets combined with energy restriction, and low fat diets alone (where 30% or less of total daily energy is derived from fat). However, there is conflicting evidence regarding their relative effectiveness.

There is conflicting evidence regarding the effectiveness of increased fibre intake.

Physical activity

Only one systematic review (NIH, 1998) has examined the effectiveness of physical activity alone for the treatment of adult obesity and overweight. Two systematic reviews (NHS CRD, 1997; NIH, 1998) considered diet and physical activity interventions. However, while reporting that physical activity alone, diet alone, and physical activity combined with diet were effective interventions in their own right, these reviews were primarily concerned with their relative effectiveness.

There is evidence that:

- Increased physical activity is effective in producing a modest total weight loss. However, diet alone was more effective than exercise alone
- Physical activity alone, diet alone, and physical activity and diet combined are effective interventions.

There is conflicting evidence regarding the relative effectiveness of physical activity combined with diet versus diet alone or physical activity alone.

Behavioural and/or cognitive therapy techniques

Behavioural therapy comprises any method to generate change in eating habits or lifestyle, including formal cognitive behaviour modification and training in behavioural skills. Cognitive therapy is also concerned with the modification of behaviour. The main principles of this treatment approach include the modification of current behaviour patterns, new adaptive learning,problem solving and a collaborative relationship between client and therapist. Cognitive therapy may be performed as part of standard behavioural therapy.

Three systematic reviews examined the effectiveness of behavioural therapy (which is usually used to support other weight loss components such as diet and physical activity) (NHS CRD, 1997; NIH, 1998; Douketis et al.,1999).

- There is evidence that a combination of behavioural therapy techniques in conjunction with other weight loss approaches is effective for the treatment of adult obesity over a one-year period.

Currently, there is limited evidence of effectiveness that supports:

- Extending the length of behavioural therapy
- Group behavioural therapy
- Correspondence courses
- Provision of structured meal plans and grocery lists
- The cognitive therapy technique of cue avoidance (individuals are asked to reduce their exposure to certain foods by making various changes to their habits)
- Cognitive rehearsal (rehearsing one's thoughts and behaviours prior to a potentially difficult situation, and planning healthy adaptive responses). There is conflicting evidence on the effectiveness of involving spouses.

Intra-abdominal fat
Intra-abdominal fat is centrally distributed within the abdominal cavity and is associated with greater health risk. Only one systematic review (NIH, 1998) has investigated the impact of a range of interventions (increased physical activity, low calorie diets and behavioural therapy) on intra-abdominal fat (as part oftotal weight loss and not as a site-specific benefit).

- There is evidence that low calorie diets are effective in decreasing intra-abdominal fat. The intra-abdominal fat loss occurs as part of total weight loss and is not a site-specific benefit
- Currently, there is limited evidence that increased physical activity is effective in reducing intra-abdominal fat in adults.

Maintenance of weight loss in adults
Obese individuals who have successfully lost weight are prone to relapse. The NIH (1998) report describes the maintenance of a lower body weight as a 'major challenge', and all weight loss approaches should be followed by a weight maintenance phase to reduce the possibility of weight regain.

Two systematic reviews (NHS CRD, 1997;Fogelholm and Kukkonen-Harjula, 2000) have examined the effectiveness of weight loss maintenance approaches.

Currently, there is limited evidence on the positiveeffects of:

- Self-help peer groups with therapist-led booster sessions on weight loss maintenance
- Daily weight charting on weight loss maintenance.

There is conflicting or inconclusive evidence regarding the effectiveness of:

- Formula diet preparations in the maintenance of weight loss
- Standard or pre-packaged foods in the maintenance of weight loss
- Increased physical activity (1,500-2,000 kilocalories per week) for weight loss maintenance
- Continued therapist contact for weight loss maintenance.

Currently, there is a lack of evidence for the effectiveness of weight focus and skills focus programmes for the maintenance of weight loss. These consisted of monthly meetings providing training in dietary and exercise behaviours compatible with maintaining weight loss (skills focus), or discussing weight loss maintenance progress and addressing difficulties using a non-specific problem solving strategy (weight focus).

Comprehensive interventions in adults
The NHS CRD (1997) review examined 11 comprehensive interventions where treatment and maintenance were combined in one intervention.

Currently, there is limited evidence to support the following strategies for weight treatment and maintenance:

- Continued therapist contact when combined with behavioural therapy and relapse prevention training
- Continued therapist contact by mail and telephone.

There is inconclusive evidence about the effectiveness of involving spouses. Currently, there is a lack of evidence to support the use of spaced versus massed booster sessions.

Settings

Worksite health promotion programmes

Two systematic reviews were identified (Hennrikus and Jeffery, 1996; Shephard, 1996) which examined the use of worksite settings for the treatment of obesity and overweight. Due to the short-term nature of these studies, the findings should be treated with caution.

- There is evidence to support the use of worksite health promotion programmes for the treatment of obesity and overweight in adults. Positive programme factors include regular participation, intensity of the intervention, associated dieting, supervision of exercise and supplementation of the exercise programme with outreach, personal counselling and plant reorganisation.

Healthcare settings and the role of health professionals

Three systematic reviews (NHS CRD, 1997; NIH, 1998; Harvey et al., 2001) have examined the effectiveness of healthcare settings or considered health professionals' management of obesity and overweight.

There is evidence to support improving the role of health professionals in the management of obesity and overweight, in particular by:

- Reminders to GPs to prescribe diets
- A brief educational training intervention on obesity management delivered by behavioural psychologists to GPs
- Encouraging shared care between GPs and a hospital service
- Use of inpatient obesity treatment services
- Training for both health professionals and leaders of self-help weight loss clinics.

APPENDIX E

The effectiveness of public health interventions for increasing physical activity among adults

(Hillsdon et al., 2004) NHS, Health Development Agency

Healthcare settings

- Review-level evidence suggests that brief advice from a doctor based in primary care, supported by written materials, is likely to be effective in producing a modest, short-term (6-12 weeks) effect on physical activity.
- Review-level evidence suggests that brief interventions, with apparently healthy individuals, based in primary care and other healthcare settings, are unlikely to be effective in producing longer-term (>8 months) changes in physical activity.
- Review-level evidence suggests there is some evidence that referral to an exercise specialist based in the community can lead to longer-term (>8 months) changes in physical activity.
- Review-level evidence suggests there is equivocal evidence for the effectiveness of interventions based in hospital outpatient clinics settings.
- Review-level evidence suggests that the short-term effectiveness of brief interventions with apparently healthy individuals with undiagnosed illness is associated with single factor interventions (physical activity only), which focus on the promotion of moderate intensity physical activity (typically walking) in a sedentary population.
- Currently there is no review-level evidence of the effectiveness of exercise referral schemes.

Community settings

- Review-level evidence suggests that community based interventions targeting individuals are effective in producing short-term changes in physical activity.
- Review-level evidence suggests that community based interventions targeting individuals are likely to be effective in producing mid- to long-term changes in physical activity.
- Review-level evidence suggests that interventions based on theories of behaviour change, which teach behavioural skills, and that are tailored to individual needs, are associated with longer-term changes in behaviour.
- Review-level evidence suggests that interventions that promote moderate intensity physical activity, particularly walking, and are not facility dependent, are also associated with longer-term changes in behaviour.
- Review-level evidence suggests that studies that incorporate regular contact with an exercise specialist tend to report sustained changes in physical activity.

Workplace settings

- Currently there is no review-level evidence of the effectiveness of workplace interventions to promote physical activity.

Older adults (50+)

- Review-level evidence suggests that interventions designed specifically for adults aged 50+ are effective in producing short-term changes in physical activity.
- Review-level evidence suggests that interventions designed specifically for adults aged 50+ are likely to be effective in producing mid- to long-term changes in physical activity.
- Review-level evidence suggests that interventions that use behavioural or cognitive approaches with a combination of group- and home-based exercise sessions rather than a class- or group-only format are associated with longer-term changes in behaviour.
- Review-level evidence suggests that interventions that promote moderate and non-endurance physical activities (eg flexibility exercises) are associated with long-term changes in behaviour.
- Review-level evidence suggests that interventions that use telephone support and follow-up are also associated with long-term behaviour change.

Adults from black and ethnic minority groups

- Currently there is no review-level evidence of the effectiveness of interventions focusing on people from ethnic minorities. Very few studies have been conducted with this target group.

Adults with physical limitations

- Currently there is no review-level evidence of the effectiveness of interventions focusing on people with physical limitations (arthritis, low back pain, chronic obstructive pulmonary disease and cystic fibrosis).